Transforming Healthcare with Qualitative Research

Drawing on the knowledge and experiences of world-renowned scientists and healthcare professionals, this important book brings together academic, medical and health systems accounts of the impact of applying qualitative research methods to transform healthcare behaviours, systems and services. It demonstrates the translation of tried-and-tested and new interventions into high-quality care delivery, improved patient pathways and enhanced systems management. It melds social theory, health systems analysis and research methods to address real-life healthcare issues in a rich and realistic fashion.

The systems and services examined include those affecting patient care and patient and professional wellbeing, and the roles and responsibilities of people providing and receiving care. Some chapters delve deeply into the human psyche, examining the very private face of health and illness. Others concentrate on public health and how people's needs can be met through health promotion and new investments. From real-time case studies to narratives on illness to theories of change, there is something here for everybody. Transforming health systems needs ingenuity – and the drive of individuals, the staying power of systems and above all the involvement of patients.

Full of novel ideas and innovative solutions from around the world, all underpinned by qualitative methods and methodologies, this book is a key contribution for advanced students, practitioners and academics interested in health services research, research methods and the sociology of health and illness.

Frances Rapport is Professor of Health Implementation Science at Macquarie University's Centre for Healthcare Resilience and Implementation Science and holds an Honorary Chair as Professor of Qualitative Health Research at Swansea University's Medical School, UK. She currently leads a team of Implementation Scientists examining new models that can successfully underpin the translation of research outcomes into practical solutions to improve healthcare service delivery.

Jeffrey Braithwaite is the Founding Director of the Australian Institute of Health Innovation; Director of the Centre for Healthcare Resilience and Implementation Science; and Professor of Health Systems Research, Faculty of Medicine, Health and Human Sciences, Macquarie University, Sydney, Australia. He is President Elect of the International Society for Quality in Health Care and a member of multiple groups of the World Health Organisation and the OECD as well as holding visiting professorships and international senior fellowships in six other Universities and think tanks in Europe and Japan.

Routledge Studies in Health and Social Welfare

For more information about this series, please visit: www.routledge.com/

Transforming Healthcare with Qualitative Research

Edited by Frances Rapport and
Jeffrey Braithwaite

Routledge
Taylor & Francis Group

LONDON AND NEW YORK

First published 2021
by Routledge
2 Park Square, Milton Park, Abingdon, Oxon OX14 4RN

and by Routledge
52 Vanderbilt Avenue, New York, NY 10017

Routledge is an imprint of the Taylor & Francis Group, an informa business

British Library Cataloguing-in-Publication Data
A catalogue record for this book is available from the British Library

Library of Congress Cataloging-in-Publication Data
A catalog record for this book has been requested

ISBN: 978-0-367-28128-1 (hbk)
ISBN: 978-0-429-29979-7 (ebk)

Typeset in Goudy
by Apex CoVantage, LLC

Contents

Boxes

Figures

Tables

Contributors

Takeru Abe is Assistant Professor at the Advanced Critical Care and Emergency Center, working also in the Department of Quality and Safety in Healthcare, at Yokohama City University Medical Center. He completed his PhD in Medical Science at the Graduate School of Medical Science, Kyushu University. His research interests include quantitative and mixed methodology, text-mining, and modelling of measurements in quality and safety in healthcare.

David C Aron is Director of Clinical Program Research and Education at the Cleveland VA Medical Center. He is a clinical endocrinologist, health services researcher and leader of the VA Quality Scholars Fellowship Program. He is Professor of Medicine and Epidemiology and Biostatistics at the School of Medicine, Case Western Reserve University, and Adjunct Professor of Organizational Behavior at the Weatherhead School of Management. Current research interests include health services and implementation research related to quality measurement and improvement and applications of principles of complex systems.

Hanna Augustsson is an affiliated researcher at Medical Management Centre, Karolinska Institutet and an Honorary Postdoctoral Fellow at Australian Institute of Health Innovation, Macquarie University. Her research interests include implementation and evaluation of organizational changes, particularly in the context of health and social care. She also works at the Unit for Implementation and Evaluation, Center for Epidemiology and Community Medicine in Stockholm Region, consulting on implementation and evaluation for public health organizations.

Elizabeth Austin is a Postdoctoral Research Fellow at the Australian Institute of Health Innovation, Macquarie University, Australia. She has a background in cognitive sciences, specialising in verbal and nonverbal communication. Dr Austin's current research is in the application of complexity science to healthcare using social psychological theories to understand resilient sociotechnical systems.

Stephanie Best is a Senior Research Fellow with the Australian Institute of Health Innovation and the Murdoch Children's Research Institute. She is a Chartered

Physiotherapist, currently engaged in implementation projects, from community engagement to health systems barriers and enablers, to implementation of genomics. She has interests in integrated teamworking and professional identity, across professional and organizational boundaries.

Mia Bierbaum is a Research Officer, tutor and PhD candidate at the Australian Institute of Health Innovation, Macquarie University, Australia. She is an experienced qualitative and quantitative researcher and skilled focus group facilitator and interviewer. Her recent research examines clinician attitudes to clinical practice guidelines in oncology, and barriers and facilitators to cochlear implant uptake in older Australians. Her interests include implementation science, health service utilization, public health promotion and the prevention of chronic disease.

Nicky Britten is Professor of Applied Health Care Research at the University of Exeter Medical School, UK. She is a medical sociologist with a long-standing interest in lay perspectives of medicines, patient-doctor communication about prescribing, management of chronic illness, qualitative synthesis and user involvement in research.

Kate Churruca is a Postdoctoral Research Fellow in the Australian Institute of Health Innovation, Macquarie University, Australia. Her research examines the complex interactions between individual, organizational and social factors in healthcare delivery, particularly how sensemaking among healthcare professionals and patients impacts on behaviour and outcomes.

Robyn Clay-Williams is a Senior Research Fellow and specialist in health systems research. She works in the field of human factors and resilient healthcare at the Australian Institute of Health Innovation, Macquarie University with expertise in human factors and resilience engineering. She develops cross-industry theoretical frameworks to describe system level behaviour and human contributions to safety in complex systems.

Ellen S Deutsch is an experienced pediatric otolaryngologist and Patient Safety and Simulation expert, with a demonstrated history of developing engaging programmes to improve skills and behaviours in individuals, teams and healthcare systems. She serves as Senior Scientist at the Children's Hospital of Philadelphia (CHOP) and Adjunct Associate Professor at the University of Pennsylvania Perelman School of Medicine. She has been Editor of the Pennsylvania Patient Safety Advisory, and Director of PeriOperative Simulation at CHOP.

Louise A Ellis is a Research Fellow at the Australian Institute of Health Innovation, Macquarie University, Australia. Her current work in health systems research is focused on complexity science and the changing nature of health systems. Dr Ellis has previously worked at The Australian Council for Educational Research and at the Brain and Mind Centre, University of Sydney, examining the use of technology to improve mental health and wellbeing in young people.

Mona Faris is a Research Officer at the Psycho-Oncology Co-Operative Research Group (PoCoG), School of Psychology, Faculty of Science, University of Sydney, Australia. She has expertise in implemtentation science working within a cluster-randomized controlled trial implementing a clinical pathway for anxiety and depression in cancer patients. Prior to joining PoCoG, she supported an examination of refractory epilsepy patient transitions through healthcare.

Dayane M C Ferreira received her qualifications in Industrial Engineering from the Universidade Federal de Juiz de Fora and Universidade Federal do Rio Grande do Sul, Brazil. She has experience in research and outreach and has provided executive training courses and consulting to both healthcare and manufacturing companies. Her areas of interest are lean production, production planning and control and healthcare management.

Emilie Francis-Auton is a Postdoctoral Research Fellow at the Australian Institute of Health Innovation, Macquarie University, Australia. She is a medical sociologist, researching social interactions and healthcare systems using qualitative methods and social theory. Her ethnographic research examines how Australian medical students are taught to navigate their relations and interactions with patients during intimate examinations.

Arthur Frank is Professor Emeritus at the University of Calgary, Canada. He studies representations of illness and suffering, examining the stories of patients and care providers, and the ethical importance of first-person narration. His work on the study of narratives has become seminal in the medical humanities. Arthur is an elected Fellow of the Royal Society of Canada and winner of the lifetime achievement award from the Canadian Bioethics Society.

Erik Hollnagel is Professor at the Institute of Regional Health Research, University of Southern Denmark; Senior Professor at Jönköping University (Sweden); Visiting Professor at the Centre for Healthcare Resilience and Implementation Science, Macquarie University (Australia); and Professor Emeritus at the Department of Computer Science, University of Linköping (Sweden). He is a leading expert in industrial safety, resilience engineering and modelling large-scale socio-technical systems.

Klay Lamprell is a researcher and writer whose work supports and examines narrative methods in medical and health services research. Dr Lamprell is a Post-Doctoral Research Fellow at the Australian Institute of Health Innovation, Macquarie University, Australia. Her current research examines experiences of illness, patient-hood and medical practice narrated in online autobiographical accounts, and descriptive discourse in doctor-patient communication.

Holly J Lanham is Associate Professor of Medicine at The University of Texas Health San Antonio. Her primary research focuses on topics intersecting information technology and human behaviour in healthcare organizations. She enjoys being part of large qualitative field studies and applying ideas from complexity science and complex adaptive systems to challenging topics.

Luci K Leykum is Professor of Medicine and Associate Chair for Clinical Innovation in the Department of Medicine at Dell Medical School at The University of Texas at Austin. She is also a Clinician-Investigator in the South Texas Veterans Health Care System and the Center Lead for the Elizabeth Dole Center of Excellence for Veteran and Caregiver Research. Her research has focused on the application of complexity science to clinical systems, examining relationships and sensemaking between providers, patients and families, and association with patient outcomes.

Janet C Long is a Health Systems Researcher with interests and expertise in knowledge translation, implementation science, and social and professional networks. She has a clinical background as a registered nurse and a science background in ecology including laboratory experience. This unique combination of clinical, science and health services research makes her a powerful connector across the translational gap between research and practice.

Zeyad Mahmoud is a multidisciplinary researcher, lecturer and course coordinator. He was a Cotutelle PhD candidate in Management Accounting and Health Innovation at both Macquarie University and the University of Nantes. For his PhD, Zeyad was leading a transdisciplinary multinational project at the intersection of management accounting, health systems research and Big History.

Elise McPherson has a Master's degree in health services research, focusing on the implementation of genomic medicine in multidisciplinary clinical settings. Her research experience spans health system implementation and sustainability, auditory neuroscience and English literature. Recently, she has moved into secondary education and is currently working as an English and Science teacher in Sydney's south-west.

Kazue Nakajima is Director and Professor of the Department of Clinical Quality Management, Osaka University Hospital, Japan. Her department serves as secretariat for Patient Safety Alliance of 45 national university hospitals and organizes annual patient safety seminars across university hospitals in Japan. Dr Nakajima has been awarded competitive research grants and prizes for safety-related activities including a hospital-wide patient engagement program.

Shin Nakajima is trained in neurosurgery. Dr Nakajima was also trained in anaesthesiology, radiology and emergency medicine. He conducted research on image-guided neurosurgery at Brigham and Women's Hospital in Boston. He currently works at Osaka National Hospital in Japan as Director of the Department of General Medicine and Deputy Director of the Department of Neurosurgery. He is dedicated to clinical education for medical students, residents and other healthcare professionals.

Kyota Nakamura works in Emergency Medicine and Intensive Care. He is Associate Professor of the Department of Patient Safety and Quality Improvement at Yokohama City University Medical Center, Japan. He works at the Advanced

Critical Care and Emergency Center of the hospital, committing himself to education for medical students and healthcare professionals. His specific interests include resuscitation, airway and ventilator management, trauma systems, disaster medicine, dynamic team performance and medical simulation training.

Mary D Patterson is a pediatric emergency medicine physician and the Associate Dean of Experiential Learning and the Lou Oberndorf Professor of Healthcare Technology at the University of Florida where she directs the Center for Experiential Learning and Simulation. She currently serves on the Board of Directors for the International Pediatric Simulation Society. Her primary research interests are in the use of medical simulation to improve patient safety, team performance and human factors work related to patient safety.

Jacqueline A Pugh is an internist, Health Services Researcher and Professor at the University of Texas Health San Antonio School of Medicine. She is currently Associate Chief of Staff for Research at the South Texas Veterans Health Care System with research interests in chronic disease management and organizational culture and improvement. She has studied how complex adaptive system theory may be a useful lens for improving healthcare quality and currently investigates sensemaking and prevention of readmissions.

Nigel Rapport is Professor of Anthropological and Philosophical Studies at the University of St. Andrews, Scotland. He is also Founding Director of the St Andrews Centre for Cosmopolitan Studies. He has held the Canada Research Chair in Globalization, Citizenship and Justice at Concordia University of Montreal, and he has been elected a Fellow of the Royal Society of Edinburgh and of the Learned Society of Wales.

Tarcisio A Saurin is Associate Professor at the Industrial Engineering Department of the Federal University of Rio Grande do Sul, Brazil. His main research interests are related to the modelling and management of complex sociotechnical systems, lean production and resilience engineering. He has carried out research and consulting projects on these topics in healthcare, construction, electricity distribution and manufacturing.

Patti Shih is a Research Fellow at the Australian Centre for Health Engagement, Evidence & Values, School of Health & Society, University of Wollongong, Australia. She is a medical sociologist, researching the intersections of health, culture and social change. She has conducted research examining the social experience of refractory epilepsy surgical treatment with patients and clinicians. She currently leads on projects using deliberative and qualitative methods in overdiagnosis and consumer health wearables.

Andrew C Sparkes is Professor of Sport, Physical Activity & Leisure in the Carnegie School of Sport at Leeds Beckett University in the UK. His research and pedagogical interests are inspired by a continuing fascination with the ways in which people experience and come to understand different forms of embodiment over time in a variety of contexts – often not of their own making.

Natalie Taylor is a health psychologist and implementation scientist with expertise in health and organizational behaviour change. Based in the Cancer
Research Division at Cancer Council New South Wales (NSW) and leading
the Behavioural and Implementation Research and Evaluation group, her
research currently focusses on testing the impact and cost-effectiveness of different approaches for translating evidence into clinical practice to improve
healthcare delivery and outcomes for patients.

Foreword

Transforming Healthcare with Qualitative Research, edited by Frances Rapport and Jeffrey Braithwaite, is a unique synthesis of 19 chapters of thought-provoking work, from some of the world's most renowned healthcare writers, encompassing *Ideas*, *Systems* and *Solutions* to healthcare problems in the twenty-first century. Academics, clinicians and systems-thinkers, at the cutting-edge of their field, pose medical, sociological and philosophical problems for readers to sink their teeth into and offer solutions to suit the needs of a global populace.

By doing so, authors pit their qualitative wits against a number of the most challenging and searching questions we have to face as we attempt to understand the current climate of healthcare development and delivery. These are challenges that are affected by scarce healthcare resources, hospitals and community settings under pressure, and with some diseases becoming ever-more resistant to treatments, putting patients' and healthcare systems' resilience under threat. The authors of this book share a single voice as they ask: How can we effectively transform our healthcare services and systems to meet the needs of a growing, aging population, on a global scale?

The book is both novel and significant, especially given the immense difficulty of putting robust qualitative work into the top-tier peer-reviewed journals. Such resistance creates *methodological myopia*, which in turn prevents new ideas from becoming more visible at scale: ideas about more democratic decision-making, how to support people in their 'adversarial struggle' of leaving the land of well to inhabit the land of the ill, how to learn using simulation, how to embrace Hollnagel's resilience grid to make care safer and how to use soft systems methodology to improve practice. And a host of other groundbreaking ideas.

For while the topic areas are extensive – from genomics to epilepsy, and from melanoma to spinal cord injury; and the methods various – from walking methods to surveys, and from narratives to interviews; it clearly reads as a single piece: a tale of others' tales, with beginnings, middles and ends. In this way, while some authors concentrate on theory-development, and others write about research conduct, and still others the challenges of implementing research findings, the chapters are grounded in what makes us tick as human beings.

I would urge you to get to know the methods and ideas contained in this book. You will find authors who care deeply about modern day healthcare services, personal wellbeing, and how to deal with systems successes and failures. At the same time if you want to consider disease presentation, disease management or clinical teamwork including how teams function through shared decision-making, by forming 'huddles', or simulating patient scenarios this book should meet your needs, offering choice examples of resilient and less resilient systems, all affected by human factors.

I commend the editors, the authors and the publishers who had the courage of conviction to back this book. It has paid off, paving the way towards forward-thinking research.

Glyn Elwyn, The Dartmouth Institute

Acknowledgements

The editors would like to acknowledge the close support of Tayhla Ryder who worked so professionally with us to edit, format and prepare the manuscript for submission. We would also like to thank Caroline Proctor for her keen eye in indexing and reading chapters, while Meagan Warwick, Tahlia Theodorou, Kristiana Ludlow, Sarah Hatem, Jackie Mullins and Sue Christian-Hayes helped search the literature, provide information to enrich some of the chapters and read sections of the book. We acknowledge the support of Zeyad Mahmood, Mitchell Sarkies, Kate Gibbons and Kelly Nguyen in proof reading parts of the finished product and considering all manner of formatting and style issues. Indeed, without the collaboration of members of the Australian Institute of Health Innovation at Macquarie University, including those based in the Centre for Healthcare Resilience and Implementation Science (CHRIS), writing and editing this book would have been a much less enjoyable task. We thank all of those at Routledge Publishing for backing this project, and we would like to extend our greatest thanks to all the authors involved. Their fascinating topics, methodological insights and health stories make the world a richer place.

Abbreviations

ADC	Automated dispensing cabinet
CAS	Complex adaptive system
CECT	Contrast-enhanced computed tomography
CFIR	Consolidated Framework for Implementation Research
CHD	Congenital heart disease
COM.B	Capability, Opportunity, and Motivation framework for Behaviour
CT	Computed tomography
DVT	Deep vein thrombosis
ECW	Everyday Clinical Work
ED	Emergency department
FRAM	Functional Resonance Analysis Method
GP	General practitioner
HCAHPS	Hospital Consumer Assessment of Healthcare Providers and Systems
HCP	Healthcare professional
IT	Information technology
LTPA	Leisure-time physical activity
NHS	National Health Services
NSF	National Service Framework
NSW	New South Wales
OR	Operating room
OT	Operating theatre
PAD	Preparation and administration of drugs
PAM	Purposeful Activity Model
QES	Qualitative evidence synthesis
QLR	Qualitative longitudinal research
RAG	Resilience Assessment Grid
RCA	Root Cause Analysis
RCT	Randomized controlled trial
SCI	Spinal cord injury
SOP	Standard Operating Procedure
SSM	Soft Systems Methodology
TEC	Tertiary Epilepsy Centre

TNM	Tumor, Node, Metastasis staging system
UK	United Kingdom
US	United States
WAD	Work-as-done
WAI	Work-as-imagined

Part 1

Ideas

We begin the substantive chapters of the book with Part 1, Ideas, which sets the scene for what is to follow. It takes both a philosophical and theoretical approach to the search for dependable qualitative evidence underpinning medical and health services research.

We open with an examination in Chapter 2 where Nicky Britten supports the transformation and resilience of healthcare systems by combining evidence synthesis with real world patient experience. Then in Chapter 3, Nigel Rapport examines the relationship between consciousness and the individual embodiment of health and illness. Coming to Chapter 4, Arthur Frank discusses the symbiotic relationship between people and their health and illness stories. Completing a tetralogy of wisdom about patients and individuals, in Chapter 5, Andrew C Sparkes takes the reader on a journey to discover how useful narratives are, as a qualitative mechanistic tool, but also as a way of mapping people's life pathways as they come to terms with life altering disease.

Building on this, but changing the pace somewhat, Frances Rapport and Jeffrey Braithwaite in Chapter 6 discuss what we call the third and fourth research paradigms. While others have written about the Third Research Paradigm in terms of corroborative data from mixed methods studies, the Fourth Research Paradigm is quite new. It concludes this section and paves the way for Part 2, Systems, by acting as a bridge between the two, and by framing the book in terms of the integral nature of theory to research to implementation, examining how rigorous planned qualitative studies drive research designs that in turn allow researchers to work alongside those at the forefront of healthcare delivery in the twenty-first century. Chapter 6 presents new approaches to data collection and analysis, particularly concentrating on 'mobile methods'; where a wide array of data are collected 'on the hoof', and where researchers work side-by-side with research participants, in active and passive roles, examining not only what they are doing, but also who they perceive themselves to be, through observations and responses to others' needs and experiences. By working alongside others on an equal footing, the fourth research paradigm encourages an assessment of what motivates actions and reactions from healthcare professionals, patients and others, while researchers are careful to work 'with', not 'on', research participants.

1 Introduction

Why this book?

Frances Rapport and Jeffrey Braithwaite

This book features an exciting collection of writings from world-renowned international academics working in the field of medicine and qualitative health research. The book has been purposefully crafted as highly interdisciplinary, with contributions from health services researchers, healthcare professionals, social scientists, anthropologists, psychologists and sociologists, to ensure wide-ranging perspectives on the topic of transforming healthcare using qualitative research methods. The authors' expertise spans policy, healthcare systems, healthcare services, teamwork, delivery systems, individual healthcare practices and individual's aspirations for good health and wellbeing. The systems and services that are examined affect not only patient care and patient and professional safety and wellbeing, but also the roles and responsibilities people take in relation to healthcare provision and receipt, including an individual's sense of self-knowing and self-actualization.

The book delves into modern-day healthcare services, some of which are delivered according to epidemiological considerations of population need, health promotion or outcomes relevant to public health. Others are delivered according to developments in cutting-edge technologies such as the single, electronic healthcare record, and still others, according to personalized treatments and therapies, such as precision medicine. Some chapters delve deeply into the human psyche – investing in personhood, personal wellbeing and life-projects, and examining the very private face of health and illness. Through contemporary examples of people's extraordinary ability to adapt and change to changing circumstances, individual resilience is examined, particularly in the face of a debilitating, chronic illness such as cancer or epilepsy. Some writers have taken a humanist approach to the presentation of theories and ideas, while others use realist theory, critical ethnography or narrative methodology to present the latest evidence.

Authors have not been afraid to ask some deep-seated questions about what healthcare professionals, patients and members of the public should expect of modern healthcare services and systems, in terms of service availability, access and clinical outcomes. By so doing, they have also raised theoretical awareness of flaws in the design of services, some of which extend to service implementation. These chapters examine how to develop systems that are flexible and adaptable to change, how to manage fractured patient care pathways, how to enhance shared-care and shared decision-making, how to contain patient and professional expectations, how to share information with family members and other healthcare professionals, and what amounts to an appropriate engagement, within and across different healthcare sectors. As a consequence, the book offers a unique contribution to the debate on whether current healthcare transformations are delivering on their promise to benefit patients, professionals, other stakeholders and society at large.

Chapters consider how, when systems function well, patients are at the receiving end of high-quality, safe and efficacious care. They also examine how, when things go wrong and systems fail to function effectively, relationships can break down, unsafe care practices can lead to medical errors, and people's lives can be irrevocably affected. While some early chapters, particularly in Part 1, concentrate almost exclusively on how illness is 'felt' within the body, and how that precipitates the notion that we carry illness with us through our lives, others, particularly in Part 2, consider how illness stories are shared through novel narrative styles that effectively reach patients and the caring community.

The nature of this book is rich in variety, from chapters describing how to transform the healthcare system to enable people to work more safely and effectively, to those arguing that patients are individuals not disease-types. Some authors take the reader down the patient's care pathway, others contend with how complex diseases and their co-morbidities are being managed. Whatever the case, it is evident from each chapter's content and quality that the depth of the authors' subject-knowledge, as well as their integrity to their craft, is of the highest calibre.

This is an ambitious project. As editors we have attempted to marry groups of writers' narratives across disciplinary backgrounds, topic areas and methodological interests – writers employing different styles, agendas and objectives. At the same time, what holds this together as a body of work is its impressive originality and integrity, and the shared intention of all authors to develop transformative healthcare systems and services using qualitative methodologies in support of best care practices.

To keep the subject contemporary and fresh, all writers have explained the transformative healthcare challenges they are examining, the qualitative methodologies and methods they are using and the aspirations they hold dear. Many chapters include the views of healthcare professionals, patients, public members, significant others, policy developers and other stakeholders who ask searching questions about how sustainable our current healthcare system really is in the face of an ever-growing, ageing population, attempting to manage with stretched resources, and the pressures of inadequate time and space. Chapters range from those presenting data from empirical research to those offering information about a new theory or research paradigm. They are all searching for knowledge on transformation, be it in service delivery, human experience or a new paradigm shift. As a result, some chapters are highly individualistic, while others depend on shared, dialogical conversations between authors, with knowledge derived from the cross-fertilization of ideas including a precise of the current literature or position statements on a new policy drive.

The book has been designed in three parts: Part 1, Ideas; Part 2, Systems; and Part 3, Solutions. Part 1, Ideas, sets the scene for what is to follow. It takes both a philosophical and theoretical approach to the search for dependable qualitative evidence underpinning medical and health services research.

Part 2 is a departure from the theoretical and philosophical aspects of qualitative methodological development, taking some of the Ideas presented in Part 1 and examining their relationship to healthcare systems' developments. In Part 2, Systems, the systems that surround the healthcare service are all examined through a qualitative lens. In Part 2, authors concentrate variously on macro, meso and micro levels of care, paying particular attention to aspects indicated in system delivery, while considering processes and mechanisms that allow care to be provided well; such as groups of professionals working together, and less well; for example, individual healthcare practitioners working in isolation.

In Part 3, Solutions, the book moves from 'ideas about health and personhood' in Part 1, and 'notions for change' in Part 2, to 'positive change'. Part 3 examines new frameworks for change management and the management of uncertainty. Together, Parts 1 to 3 offer a unique and highly creative reflection on the current values and credibility of qualitative methods within medicine, health services research and health systems research. Methods are examined for their versatility and rigour, while writers are bold in predicting where new methodologies might take us in our search for sustainable, high-quality, safe systems of care that serve personal preferences and needs. Seen holistically, chapters celebrate the perspicacity and drive of individuals: those who are sick and those who are well, those who care for others and those who are cared-for, those who write policy and those who implement policy, those who research and those being researched. Together they provide a clear vision for the future of qualitative research methods in this field, while examining what is being researched and what needs to be researched more. Together they reveal the qualitative tools at our disposal and those that can only be imagined, to drive research forward towards implementable interventions, proclaiming a chance to improve healthcare systems worldwide, in ways that are both transactional and realistic, for the good of society.

2 Qualitative evidence synthesis and conceptual development

Nicky Britten

Introduction

Research in healthcare often addresses practical problems about best treatments for specific health problems or the best ways of providing healthcare to particular groups of people. Since the 1990s healthcare research has been in thrall to evidence-based medicine and its associated hierarchy of evidence. Randomized controlled trials are considered the best method for establishing the efficacy of drugs and other treatments. In this context, qualitative research is considered to be inferior due to its inability to provide precise quantitative estimates, its small sample sizes, its supposed lack of generalizability and its 'anecdotal' nature. However, healthcare research has to achieve much more than identify best treatments. Even solutions to practical problems require underpinning mechanisms or theoretical explanations. In this chapter, I aim to show how the synthesis of qualitative evidence can provide conceptual insights which have the potential to improve and transform the quality of healthcare.

Background and problem

Although qualitative research has a rich and distinguished history in the social sciences, qualitative researchers have struggled to get their work taken seriously in medical research. Reviewers of papers sent to medical journals in the 1990s criticized qualitative research as being 'anecdotal' due to their small sample sizes. This began to change with the publication of a series of papers about different aspects of qualitative research in the *British Medical Journal* in 1995. These were later republished as an edited book which is now going into its fourth edition, suggesting a sustained appetite for an introductory text aimed at medical researchers (Pope and Mays 2006). Over time, qualitative research has become more acceptable as evidenced by growing numbers of qualitative papers in many medical journals. But 20 years after the original series, the *British Medical Journal* stated that qualitative research papers were an extremely low priority, claiming that qualitative papers were less highly cited than quantitative papers. This was despite the fact that of the 20 most influential papers published in the *British Medical Journal* over the previous 20 years, the top three qualitative papers were more highly cited than the top three randomized controlled trials (RCTs) (Greenhalgh et al. 2016). In advocating the value of qualitative research, it would be misguided to overlook the shortcomings of some published papers, or to avoid talking about how the quality of qualitative research could be improved. The development of methods of qualitative evidence synthesis (QES) was driven in part by the need to address some of the shortcomings of primary qualitative research. These problems included the publication of many small-scale studies in limited populations coupled with the lack of citation of similar or relevant previous research, which impeded the building of a cumulative knowledge base. Many of these primary studies were descriptive with little or no conceptualization, and thus limited transferability or generalizability. Consequently, qualitative evidence synthesis can be seen as a way of enhancing the contribution of qualitative research to healthcare, with its emphasis on credibility as well as transferability.

Pathways to addressing the problem

In this chapter I will focus on one method of qualitative evidence synthesis, namely meta-ethnography (Noblit and Hare 1988). It is one of the most widely used methods of QES. It uses explanations, theories or concepts as building blocks with the aim of producing conceptual innovation. Studies which are purely descriptive make little contribution to meta-ethnography (Campbell et al. 2012). By bringing together the results of several small-scale studies, qualitative synthesis can add to the weight of evidence.

Primary qualitative research can contribute to the transformation of health services by engaging with the views and experiences of those receiving and providing healthcare. Much of this work reveals the differing and sometimes conflictual perspectives of patients and professionals. While it is hard to measure what impact primary qualitative research has had, there are two developments which provide a stronger rationale for greater understanding of patients' perspectives. The literature on complex interventions emphasizes the need to theorize why interventions do or do not work (Craig et al. 2008), and the development of theories and possible mechanisms requires an appreciation of how it feels to be on the receiving end of healthcare. Second, the growing emphasis on self-management of chronic illness also requires an understanding of how patients engage, or don't, with treatments and advice. In this more receptive landscape, QES can provide conceptual development which builds on the insights of primary research.

I will illustrate the potential of QES using five exemplar syntheses including three I co-authored (Britten et al. 2002; Pound et al. 2005; Britten and Pope 2012; Malpass et al. 2009; Toye et al. 2013) (see Box 2.1). This does not constitute the summary of a field of research but shows the transformative potential of this method. These syntheses were all concerned with patients' experiences of treatments for various long-term conditions. Each synthesis identified several concepts and produced a verbal line of argument, and three of them also produced conceptual models in the form of visual figures and diagrams. Four syntheses provided an explanation of lay decision-making and there were several recurring issues.

Some provided clear guidance for professionals; one identified the importance to patients of an often overlooked topic, the safety of medicines. They all offered "realistic insights into the everyday experiences and interactions of patients and professionals" (Rapport and Braithwaite 2018, 5). I will present three of the inter-linked concepts which emerged from one or more of these syntheses: lay testing; identity threat; and managing illness as struggle.

Box 2.1   Concepts and lines of argument identified in each synthesis

Concepts – Adherence; self-regulation; aversion to medicines; alternative coping strategies; sanctions; selective disclosure

Line of argument – "There are two distinct forms of medicine-taking: adherent medicine-taking and self-regulation. The latter reflects aversion to medicines. The use of alternative coping strategies is one expression of this aversion. In self-regulation, patients carry out their own cost-benefit analyses, informed by their own cultural meanings and resources. Thus the concept of self-regulation includes the use of alternative coping strategies. Sanctions from health professionals, such as warnings, coercion or the threat of coercion, serve to inhibit self-regulation which can only flourish if sanc-tions are not severe. There is selective disclosure in the way in which patients manage the information they give to health professionals. Patients may not articulate views of information that they do not perceive to be medically legitimated, such as their use of alternative coping strategies. Fear of sanc-tions and guilt can produce selective disclosure" (Britten et al. 2002, 213).

Concepts – Lay evaluation; medicines and identity; resistance

Line of argument – "The synthesis revealed widespread caution about taking medicines and highlighted the lay practice of testing medicines, mainly for adverse effects. Some concerns about medicines cannot be resolved by lay evaluation, however, including worries about dependence, tolerance and addiction, the potential harm from taking medicines on a long-term basis and the possibility of medicines masking other symptoms. Additionally, in some cases medicines had a significant impact on identity, presenting problems of disclosure and stigma. People were found to accept their medicines either passively or actively, or to reject them. Some were coerced into taking medicines. . . . Many modifications appeared to reflect a desire to minimize the intake of medicines and this was echoed in some peoples' use of non-pharmacological treatments to either supplant or sup-plement their medicines. Few discussed regimen changes with their doctors. We conclude that the main reason why people do not take their medicines as prescribed is not because of failings in patients, doctors or systems, but because of concerns about the medicines themselves. On the whole, the findings point to considerable reluctance to take medicine and a preference to take as little as possible. We argue that peoples' resistance to medicine taking needs to be recognized and that the focus should be on developing ways of making medicines safe, as well as identifying and evaluating the treatments that people often choose in preference to medicines" (Pound et al. 2005, 133).

Concepts – Identity; ordinariness; non-compliance; reciprocity

Line of argument – "A person with asthma's sense of identity is associated with the ways in which they perceive and use their medicines: those accepting the asthma identity will view medicines as an aid to normalization, while those not accepting this identity will view medicines as an obstacle to normalization" (Britten and Pope 2012, 54).

Concepts – Lay evaluation; medication career; moral career; decisive moral junctures [plus different selves]

Line of argument – "A patient prescribed antidepressants embarks on two journeys: the ill self negotiating the medical world and understanding the medicated self. Negotiating the medical world is labelled . . . as the 'medication career' because it is about the patient's experience of antidepressant medication and treatment decisions through their illness. Understanding the medicated self is labelled . . . the 'moral career' because it involves various 'interpretive dilemmas' in the illness career, in which ideas of self-concept as 'good' or 'bad' compete" (Malpass et al. 2009, 165).

Concept – Pain as an adversarial struggle

Line of argument – "Struggle pervades multiple levels of the person's experience, sense of body and self, biographical trajectory, reciprocal relationships, and experience of healthcare services. The struggle to keep hold of a sense of self while feeling misunderstood and not believed was described. Despite this adversarial struggle, the present model offers an understanding of how a person with chronic musculoskeletal pain can move forward alongside their pain" (Toye et al. 2013, e833).

Lay testing

The concept of lay testing was elaborated in three syntheses, the later syntheses citing the earlier ones (Britten et al. 2002; Pound et al. 2005; Malpass et al. 2009). It refers to the way in which people carry out their own evaluations of their medicines, using their own criteria, normally well away from professional oversight. The criteria informing lay testing include weighing up costs and benefits; adverse effects; evaluating the acceptability of a regimen in everyday life; weighing and balancing the impact of medicines against impact of the health condition; stopping the medicine to see what happens; observing others and obtaining information from them; and using subjective and objective indicators. Pound et al.

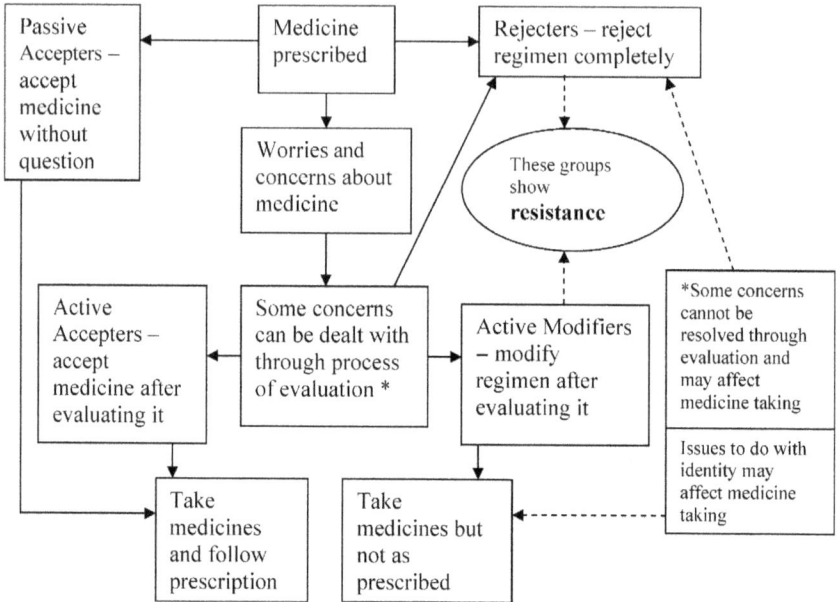

Figure 2.1 Model of medicine taking.

Source: Reprinted with permission from Elsevier: Social Science & Medicine. Pound, P, N Britten, M Morgan, L Yardley, C Pope, G Daker-White, and R Campbell. 2005. "Resisting medicines: A synthesis of qualitative studies of medicine taking." *Social Science & Medicine* 61 (1):133–155.

(2005) produced a model of medicine taking which sets out several decision pathways, depending on the outcome of lay evaluation (see Figure 2.1). Malpass et al. (2009) used the concept of lay evaluation and produced their own model of the decision-making process relevant to antidepressants. They called this process the 'medication career' in contrast to the 'moral career' simultaneously experienced by patients. The concept of lay testing is compatible with the fact that treatment effect sizes derived from RCTs are population averages, and that even 'effective treatments' will not work for everyone; this is partly due to the fact that many trials only recruit from highly selected atypical populations. The rationale for lay testing (identifying adverse effects, establishing whether the treatment works for a given individual, and finding the optimal dose) is the same rationale as for N of 1 trials. This concept of lay testing is at odds with the medicocentric concept of non-compliance (or its synonym non-adherence), which is the label given to any form of medicine taking which deviates from medical prescription.

Identity threat and stigma

Pound et al. (2005) showed how medicine use was closely related to the acceptance or non-acceptance of a person's diagnosis in the context of several conditions.

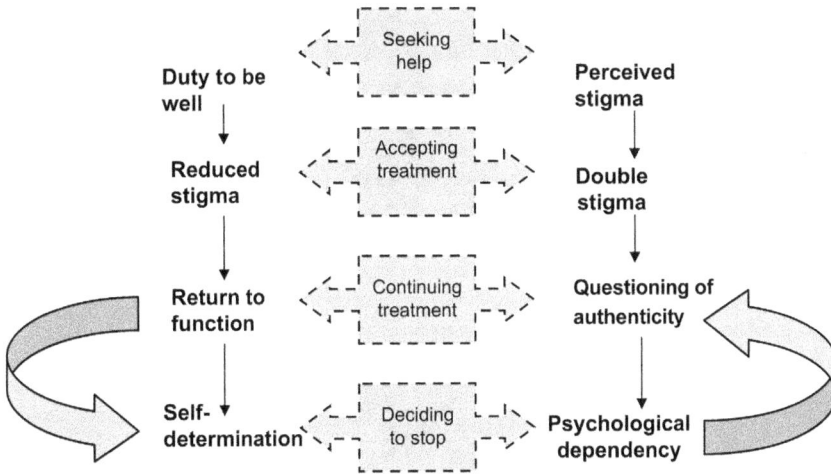

Figure 2.2 The four decisive moral junctures.

Source: Reprinted with permission from Elsevier: *Social Science & Medicine*. Malpass, A, A Shaw, D Sharp, F Walter, G Feder, M Ridd, and D Kessler. 2009. "'Medication career' or 'Moral career'? The two sides of managing antidepressants: A meta-ethnography of patients' experience of antidepressants." *Social Science & Medicine* 68:154–168.

Using the results of the same synthesis, Britten and Pope (2012) produced a line of argument to take this further in the context of asthma. Malpass et al. (2009) used the concept of moral career to describe the process by which people try to manage tensions about their identity at four moral junctures in their journey with antidepressants. These junctures, or time points, were seeking help; accepting treatment; continuing treatment; and deciding to stop treatment (see Figure 2.2). The threats to identity were the perceived stigma of mental illness; the double stigma of taking medicines for mental illness; questions of authenticity and normality; and psychological dependency on medicines. The model produced by Malpass et al. (2009) showed how the twin processes of medication career and moral career run alongside each other and contribute to the lay evaluation process. The synthesis by Toye et al. (2013) showed how people suffering chronic pain had to struggle to keep hold of a sense of self and had to reconstruct their sense of self over time.

Managing illness as struggle

The syntheses also highlighted various tensions and struggles that people grapple with in the course of managing illness and treatment. The main concept emerging from Toye et al.'s (2013) synthesis was that of an adversarial struggle (see Figure 2.3). People managing non-malignant chronic pain struggled: to affirm their sense of self; to reconstruct their sense of self over time; to construct an explanation for their suffering in the face of disbelief; to negotiate the healthcare

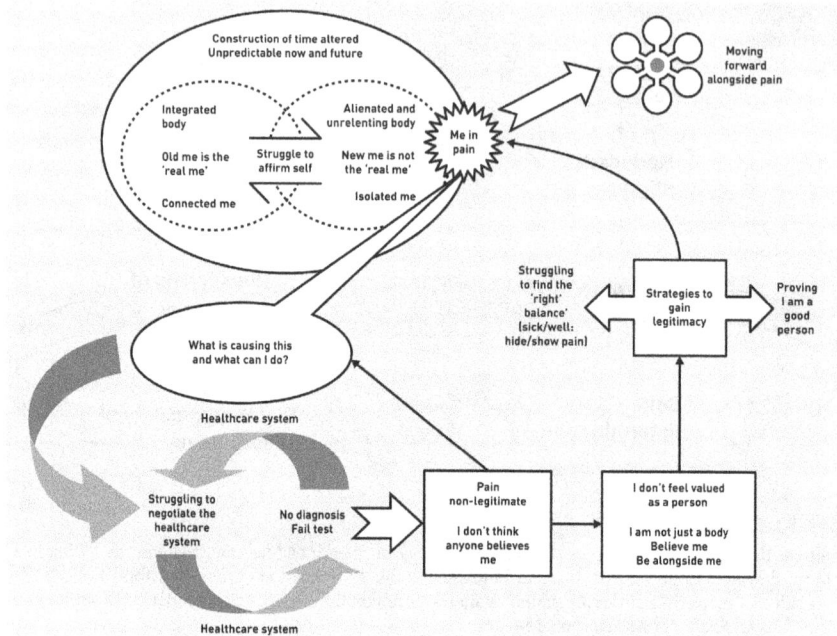

Figure 2.3 Conceptual model: A constant adversarial struggle.

Source: Toye, F, K Seers, N Allcock, M Briggs, E Carr, J Andrews, and K Barker. 2013. "Patients' experiences of chronic non-malignant musculoskeletal pain: A qualitative systematic review." *British Journal of General Practice* 63 (617):829–841. Page e834.

system; and to prove their legitimacy. Different kinds of struggles were identified by Malpass et al. (2009), resulting from the antagonist nature of the moral junctures. These were times of conflict when people were struggling with competing perceptions of social norms and competing meanings of medicines. The authors of both these syntheses provided clear guidance about how health professionals could support people caught up in such struggles, by identifying the specific nature of the struggles at different points in the patient's journey, and by understanding how they have been affected by their health condition.

Discussion

These syntheses illustrate the potential of qualitative evidence synthesis to contribute new ideas and practical suggestions which could lead to improved healthcare. The conceptual contribution of these syntheses is a deeper and innovative understanding of the perspectives of patients and the ways these differ from those of health professionals. The syntheses provide a deeper understanding of the real world experiences of patients who have to manage both their health conditions and their interactions with health professionals (Rapport and Braithwaite 2018). Although the concepts are grounded in primary research, generalizations are strengthened when concepts or explanations derive from several primary studies and apply across several health conditions.

Taking the concept of lay testing, the contrasting medicocentric ideology of compliance led to overlooking the most obvious factor in medicine taking: the medicines themselves (Pound et al. 2005). Those researching non-compliance have sought explanations in the behaviour of patients and doctors or the relationships between them. Successive Cochrane reviews about interventions to support adherence have not tended to engage with patients' own ideas or experiences and have found limited evidence of successful interventions. These reviews focus on overcoming barriers to adherence by providing education, counselling or cognitive behavioural therapy. Nieuwlaat et al. concluded that "a cure for non-adherence is nowhere to be seen", suggesting that non-adherence is comparable to a disease (Nieuwlaat et al. 2014, 18). Pound et al. point out that "the huge and unproductive literature on 'non-compliance' only exists because so many people have continued to resist taking medicines despite sustained admonishment and interventions" (Pound et al. 2005, 152). The concept of lay testing is transformational because it takes patients' perspectives seriously, instead of dismissing them as 'lay beliefs', a term which ignores the considerable dangers of prescription medicines. Earlier sociological studies of medicine taking emphasized the rationality of lay behaviour and challenged the ideology of compliance (Stimson 1974; Donovan 1995) but later authors have often adopted a medical agenda. Once the limitations of randomized controlled trials are acknowledged, and the fact that trials produce population-level estimates of effectiveness relevant to highly selected populations, the habit of lay testing may be seen as a rational response. It is also a rational response to the fact that adverse drug reactions are a significant cause of hospital admissions (Pirmohamed et al. 2004) and the fact that many new drugs are taken off the market due to safety concerns (Davis and Abraham 2013).

The transformative potential of the concepts produced by these syntheses lies in the shift of focus from the medical gaze and the 'delivery' of care to its receipt. This shift emphasizes the lifeworld of patients and carers rather than healthcare systems and professionally driven imperatives. Patients are often more concerned with managing their everyday lives than managing their biomarkers. Above all, patients seek good relationships with professionals in which they are recognized as "more than just a body" (Toye et al. 2013, 831). Recent development of the more patient-centred concept of treatment burden suggests that this change of perspective is taking hold (Dobler et al. 2018).

Qualitative research can help address the epistemic injustice embedded in healthcare, by taking patient perspectives seriously. Fricker's concept of epistemic injustice encompasses both testimonial injustice and hermeneutic injustice (Fricker 2007). Testimonial injustice occurs when someone's contribution is not believed; for example, when a patient's report of the side effect of a drug is not taken seriously. Hermeneutic injustice occurs when someone lacks the conceptual tools to understand their situation; for example, when a patient does not understand the medical terminology used in a consultation with a doctor. Qualitative research can help remedy the former injustice by giving credence and authority to patients' perspectives and explaining their relevance to the delivery of good healthcare. In relation to hermeneutical injustice, given the increasing online accessibility of academic research, it may be that the concepts produced by QES can provide patients and carers with tools to understand their own experiences. Patients' access to research may be facilitated by authors who communicate the results of their work using visual images on social media (see Figure 2.4) People who think about their own behaviour as 'lay testing' rather than disobedience may perhaps be more willing to discuss what they are doing with prescribers.

Clearly QES has its limitations. There are several challenges still to be addressed in this field, such as the need for efficient literature searching, greater patient and public involvement, more accessible outputs and active engagement with disconfirming views or refutational findings. Of the three main ways in which Noblit and Hare claimed that studies can relate to each other, only two (reciprocal translation and line of argument synthesis) have been commonly reported (Noblit and Hare 1988). The third type, refutational synthesis, is rarely if ever reported. Some studies do not fit a synthesis when they are not based in similar prior assumptions (Britten and Pope 2012) but this is not the same as refutation.

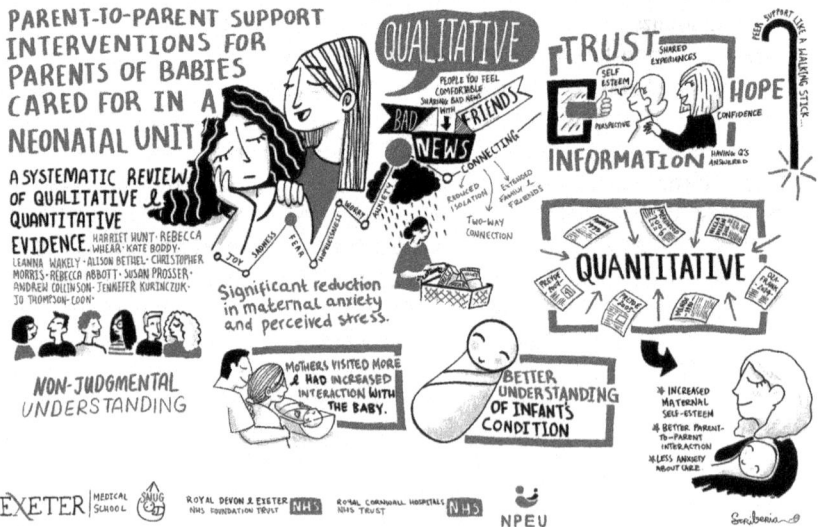

Figure 2.4 Social media representation of a systematic review.

Source: Hunt, H, R Abbott, K Boddy, R Whear, L Wakely, A Bethel, . . . J Kurinczuk. 2019. "They've walked the walk": A systematic review of quantitative and qualitative evidence for parent-to-parent support for parents of babies in neonatal care." *Journal of Neonatal Nursing* 25 (4):166–176.

Implications for practice or theory

Concepts emerging from these syntheses can provide guidance for health professionals. They may also help patients and carers understand what is happening to them by giving them new ways of thinking. Malpass et al. show practitioners the specific nature of struggles about antidepressants at particular junctures (Malpass et al. 2009). These struggles give clues about what support might be most appropriate at different junctures. At the point of accepting treatment, patients may be trying to balance the tension between reducing stigma if antidepressants are seen as correcting a physical deficiency of serotonin and increasing stigma because these medicines label the taker as having a mental illness. The concepts of lay testing and resistance to medicine could help professionals and patients open up discussions about reluctance to take medicines and promote realistic conversations about prescribing, thus promoting shared decision-making. This understanding of struggle can help identify the appropriate focus for professional support; or at least lead to an acknowledgment that there is a struggle and what the struggle is about. This enhanced understanding of, and engagement with, patients' perspectives may be seen as part of person-centred care, which involves an engagement with the person's narrative and their lifeworld (Ekman et al. 2011). The model produced by Toye et al. suggested that a central aspect of the patient's relationship with a health professional was the recognition that the patient was a person whose life had been deeply changed, for the worse, by the experience of chronic pain (Toye et al. 2013).

Conclusion

The syntheses presented in this chapter have provided new concepts which are relevant to healthcare. These concepts are potentially transformational in addressing the epistemic injustice which is inherent in much healthcare: the marginalization or dismissal of patients' perspectives and the dominance of medicocentric assumptions. These concepts illuminate the rationale behind seemingly irrational behaviour and the struggles patients are engaged in. Qualitative research has the capacity to critique the assumptions of quantitative research and to challenge taken for granted ideologies such as compliance or the safety of pharmaceutical interventions. This research also supports a person-centred approach which requires understanding of how a person's identity may be affected by illness and treatment. These insights are increasingly relevant in an era when 'self-management' is often seen as a solution to systemic problems in healthcare.

Acknowledgements

I would like to thank Dr Emma France for giving me access to some of the materials from the eMERGe project.

References

Britten, N, R Campbell, C Pope, J Donovan, M Morgan, and R Pill. 2002. "Using meta ethnography to synthesise qualitative research: A worked example." *Journal of Health Services Research & Policy* 7:209–215.

Britten, N, and C Pope. 2012. "Medicine taking for Asthma: A worked example of meta-ethnography." In *Synthesizing Qualitative Research: Choosing the Right Approach*, edited by K Hannes and C Lockwood. Oxford: John Wiley & Sons, Ltd.

Campbell, R, P Pound, M Morgan, G Daker-White, N Britten, R Pill, . . . J Donovan. 2012. "Evaluating meta-ethnography: Systematic analysis and synthesis of qualitative research." *Health Technology Assessment* 15 (43):1–164.

Craig, P, P Dieppe, S Macintyre, S Michie, I Nazareth, and M Petticrew. 2008. "Developing and evaluating complex interventions: The new medical research council guidance." *BMJ* 337 (a1655).

Davis, C, and J Abraham. 2013. *Unhealthy Pharmaceutical Regulation: Innovation, Politics and Promissory Science*. Basingstoke: Palgrave Macmillan.

Dobler, CC, N Harb, CA Maguire, CL Armour, C Coleman, and M Hassan Murad. 2018. "Treatment burden should be included in clinical practice guidelines." *BMJ* 363 (k4065).

Donovan, J. 1995. "Patient decision making: The missing ingredient in compliance research." *International Journal of Technology Assessment in Health Care* 11 (3):443–455.

Ekman, I, K Swedberg, C Taft, A Lindseth, A Norberg, E Brink, . . . K Stibrant Sunner-hagen. 2011. "Person-centered care – Ready for prime time." *European Journal of Cardiovascular Nursing* 10:248–251.

Fricker, M. 2007. *Epistemic Injustice: Power and the Ethics of Knowing*. Oxford: Oxford University Press.

Greenhalgh, T, E Annandale, R Ashcroft, J Barlow, N Black, A Bleakley, . . . S Ziebland. 2016. "An open letter to The BMJ editors on qualitative research." *BMJ* 352:i563.

Malpass, A, A Shaw, D Sharp, F Walter, G Feder, M Ridd, and D Kessler. 2009. "'Medication career' or 'Moral career'? The two sides of managing antidepressants: A meta-ethnography of patients' experience of antidepressants." *Social Science & Medicine* 68:154–168.

Nieuwlaat, R, N Wilczynski, T Navarro, N Hobson, R Jeffery, A Keepanasseril, . . . S Jack. 2014. "Interventions for enhancing medication adherence." *Cochrane Database of Systematic Reviews* (11).

Noblit, GW, and RD Hare. 1988. *Meta-Ethnography: Synthesizing Qualitative Studies*. Newbury Park: Sage.

Pirmohamed, M, S James, S Meakin, C Green, A Scott, T Walley, . . . A Breckenridge. 2004. "Adverse drug reactions as cause of admission to hospital: Prospective analysis of 18,820 patients." *BMJ* 329:15–19.

Pope, C, and N Mays. 2006. *Qualitative Research in Health Care*. 3rd ed. Oxford: Blackwell Publishing, Ltd.

Pound, P, N Britten, M Morgan, L Yardley, C Pope, G Daker-White, and R Campbell. 2005. "Resisting medicines: A synthesis of qualitative studies of medicine taking." *Social Science & Medicine* 61:133–155.

Rapport, F, and J Braithwaite. 2018. "Are we on the cusp of a fourth research paradigm? Predicting the future for a new approach to methods-use in medical and health services research." *BMC Medical Research Methodology* 18 (1):131. doi: 10.1186/s12874-018-0597-4.

Stimson, G. 1974. "Obeying doctor's orders: A view from the other side." *Social Science & Medicine* 8:97–104.

Toye, F, K Seers, N Allcock, M Briggs, E Carr, J Andrews, and K Barker. 2013. "Patients' experiences of chronic non-malignant musculoskeletal pain: A qualitative systematic review." *British Journal of General Practice* 63 (617):829–841. doi: 10.3399/bjgp13X675412.

3 The life-project of personal wellbeing

Modern healthcare and the individuality of health

Nigel Rapport

In "On Liberty", John Stuart Mill's celebrated essay from 1859, the philosopher sought to establish the principles of a liberal society based on the personal freedoms of individual citizens. The following passage in particular, I shall argue, contains much that is still relevant for contemporary healthcare, even providing a yardstick for innovative practice and transformative potential:

> The only freedom which deserves the name, is that of pursuing our own good in our own way, so long as we do not attempt to deprive others of theirs, or impede their efforts to obtain it. *Each is the proper guardian of his own health, whether bodily, or mental and spiritual.* Mankind are greater gainers by suffering each other to live as seems good to themselves, than by compelling each to live as seems good to the rest.
>
> (Mill 1909, 215 my emphasis)

Mill not only presages medicine that is personal and geared to the wellbeing of the individual body, but one that is also intrinsically private. 'Health' is a personal and also private matter, it will be urged in this chapter. There are limits to what the healthcare practitioner should endeavour to know, can expect to know and can hope to know: there are limits to how healthcare practitioners should and can practically 'engage' – administer to, appropriate – the individual body and the habits of health and wellbeing of the human Other in the role of patient (cf. Rapport 2018).

Some 100 years after Mill, Iris Murdoch argued for an understanding of 'goodness' as a social virtue in terms of restraint: refraining from visiting one's desires upon others. The 'good society', she contended (2001), as much concerned normative endeavour to *refrain from* doing others harm as it did to do others good. 'Goodness' resided in securing a kind of space in which individuals may come into their own. An institutional social order could not foresee and ought not to attempt to prescribe what 'coming into one's own' might entail in terms of the substance of an individual citizen's life. But it may still hope to afford the citizen an optimum of opportunity for its expression, and to treat that self-expression as a right. 'Goodness' was the instituting of arrangements which balanced a general inclusiveness and a universalization of rights against the particularities of individual sovereignty.

But what precisely can Mill's and Murdoch's formulations mean for modern healthcare: in the context of technologies that may outstrip the knowledge of patients; and in the context of a liberalism or civility that might now possess cosmopolitan ambitions globally to include any and every human being as citizen; and yet in the context of mass societies whose compressed populations and cultures entail a diversity of 'identities' seeking 'rightful' recognition and accommodation? There is, I shall argue, an intrinsic individuality to physical wellbeing to which healthcare in a liberal-cosmopolitan society must endeavour to do global justice and to which technological advance can increasingly contribute.

The organism-in-its-environment: earthworms and humans

From the perspective of neurology, Gerald Edelman has argued that it is through activity-in-the-world, from before birth onwards, that the brain comes not only to structure itself in a particular and personal way but also to structure, to know and form, its bodily 'hexis': its habitual bodily environment. "Each individual person [comes to be] like no other", Edelman writes (1992, 171), for each is motivated by their own historical system of physiological 'values' and gratifications: brain-plus-body-plus-environment come to form a single phenomenal unit.

In different language, this significantly echoes recent work in natural history which argues that some organisms do not so much adapt themselves to environments as create environments adapted to them. In "The Extended Organism: The Physiology of Animal-Built Structures", Scott Turner (2000) elaborates on a thesis that certain animals may change the environmental conditions in which they live to the extent that these fabrications beyond the outer extents of their bodies should nevertheless be conceived of as external organs of their physiology. For the structures mould the environment in such a way as to affect the flow of matter, energy and information through the organism as much as do as their internal bodily workings. Nor is there reason to exclude the human animal from this proposition. Indeed, human social, cultural and technological accoutrements make Turner's work even more suggestive.

Animal-built structures are ubiquitous, Turner considers, whether ephemeral in construction and duration or more lasting. Moreover, it is appropriate in certain cases at least to consider these as parts of the animals themselves, as organs of their particular physiologies: the effects of these structures are such that it would be inappropriate to delimit the identity of the organisms by the outer integument of their bodies; the animal organisms extend beyond themselves into the environments they fashion. What makes a living organism distinctive and individual, then, is not the existence of its boundary or integument per se but the nature of what a boundary does.

The boundary of an organism is best thought of as *a process* whereby certain internal conditions of life are maintained over and against external conditions or variations. Most of an organism's major physiological functions operate to provide a degree of stability or 'homeostasis' to its internal environment: the proper conditions of temperature, pH and solute concentration, and the organized delivery and distribution of nutrients, fuel, oxidant and wastes. Differently put, while the persistence of a particular organism's individual identity may be said to come about by way of the existence of a boundary between it and its environment, this boundary is in fact thoroughly permeable, causing matter and energy continually to pass through it. Furthermore, this channelling of external materials should not be envisaged as a passive process; for organisms exert adaptive control over the flows of matter and energy (thereby maintaining a homeostatic state in the face of changing conditions). Hence, by further structurally modifying their environments, organisms extend the range of homeostatic conditions necessary for their form of life from 'inside' their 'bodies' to outside. Altering the random or entropic nature of energy- and matter-flows, they impose an 'orderliness' on nature, adapting their environments to themselves – and, indeed, *as* themselves. In short, through metabolic processes, animals use energy to produce homeostatic conditions in 'external' environments that they have personally ordered into known and usable spaces – precisely as they do 'internally'. "The principles of thermodynamics do not stop at the organism's skin", Turner summarizes (2000, 7), and the environment "can [come to] have physiology" (11).

To avert briefly to one of Turner's specific examples may be to consider the construction of soil burrows by earthworms (2000, 81–119). The earthworms' purpose in doing this is a 'personal' one: to aerate and fertilize soils and so 'co-opt' these soils into acting as accessory kidneys, ensuring the worms' survival in an otherwise uninhabitable space. For earthworms evolved to be freshwater creatures. Their problem in living on land is keeping the right balance of water and salts in their bodies: maintaining a differential between the condition of the liquids inside their bodies and out, and offsetting a thermodynamic flux which would naturally tend towards equalization. Earthworms deploy their energies to change soil ecosystems: secreting mucus from their body surfaces, passing soil through their bodies (so that mucus collects to it) and defecating calcite. These three processes act against entropy: keeping burrows open, enabling the soil to absorb sufficient water, but also holding it weakly enough for earthworms to gain access to it. The result is to vastly expand the natural horizons where worms can live.

Earthworms have made a choice, Turner concludes. They have decided to change the environment rather than change themselves – evolutionarily a far faster and more flexible process – making the soil into an accessory organ that balances their bodily liquidity. As "architects and engineers of their environments", earthworms are able to effect an orderliness at a scale many times greater than their organismic integument so that their personal lives ramify broadly in time and space (Turner 2000, 7).

What kind of connection should now be made between this natural-historical thesis and a social-scientific one: between the world of the earthworm and that of human being? A standard (affirmative) reaction might be to say that culture is the human equivalent of animal-physiological constructions. Through our clothes, our houses, our systems of production, our aesthetic traditions, our systems of alliance, exchange and reciprocity, we extend our physiological genotype so as produce a sociocultural phenotype-plus-environment that enables us to co-opt the natural world to our adaptational advance. Anthropologist Amos Rapoport thus describes cultures as 'underwriting' the environments in which human beings live to the extent that these environments become material expressions of social structures. A human 'built environment' comes into being that involves organizations of "time, space, communication and meaning, add[ing] up to a complete ecological system" (Rapoport 1998, 488, 467). Here are cultures as 'non-natural' ecosystems (Tallis 2001, 4).

But alongside sociocultural spaces Rapoport also refers to the creation of 'personal space': the "movable 'bubble' of space that surrounds an individual" (1998, 486). Here, I suggest, is a way to adapt Turner's insights in a more subtle fashion: it is individual human beings and not just species or groups that may be appreciated as "architects and engineers of their environments". More precisely, the 'life-projects' of individual human beings may be seen as kinds of environmental architecture that extend control of personal identity beyond the skin, conditioning an environment in a personally adaptive way. By 'life-project' one refers, as did Edelman, to that practical history of intentioned activity-in-the-world whereby the individual human being is responsible for the co-constitution of brain-plus-body-plus-environment (Rapport 2005).

Since consciousness is inevitably individually embodied, an individual history of worldly engagement develops concerning how a person comes to interpret and give meaning to what they perceive around them. These personal 'worldviews' lead in turn to lives of particular and individual character, directionality and destination (Rapport 1993). Anthropologist Gregory Bateson spoke of the individual human being in this connection as an 'energy source' and an 'organism-in-its-environment' (1972, 426). In short, developing their own worldviews and pursuing their own life-projects may be conceived of as forms of intentional practice which procure for the individual human being an extended environmental homeostasis of a significantly personal kind.

The personal ecology of the individual life-project

It is useful to refer, very briefly, to a long philosophical history of conceptualizing 'life-projects' (from Greek Stoicism to modern Existentialism), and the links asserted between these and the nature of individual human identity. According to Epictetus, for instance, it was by virtue of possessing a personal 'life-policy' (proharus) that individuals took intellectual responsibility for their lives and might devote them to inviolable purposes of their own. Proharus, for Epictetus, bespoke an inner will – the real and true self – that no extraneous, determining force could assail. It was their personal life-policies that emancipated people from being in thrall to externalities of customary practice and convention.

While suspicious of what he saw as Epictetus's polarizations between the 'proud' life-policy of the Stoic and the 'passions' of the slave, Søren Kierkegaard shared the idea of human beings as consciously responsible for themselves – contra external circumstance – and suggested that nothing in their environment was beyond their action or challenge. Individuals should identify themselves with the 'project' of manifesting integrity and entirety in their lives, Kierkegaard adjured, and by being in possession of a knowledge of who they were and how they should be, of creating a purposive pattern. And as with Epictetus, successful self-determination was seen by Kierkegaard to derive ultimately from a quality of individual will intrinsic to human embodiment.

Equally, will was something that Friedrich Nietzsche came to emphasize in his formulation of the self-creation of human life, and it is in his hands that the individual 'life-project' receives perhaps its most intensive philosophical treatment. What Nietzsche wished to convey, particularly through his phrasing of an individual's 'will to power', was that intrinsic to the person was the possibility, even the proclivity, of a self-becoming which amounted to a continuous self-overcoming. To be a human being was perforce to 'create new things' since all acts and interpretations were entirely their own (Nietzsche 1968, 403). The individual created the perspectives or worldviews by which they identified what the world contained, including the values by which the world was assessed. But even as the energy and the creativity that were foundational of individual existence remained singular in source, there was the further impulse to will lives that were continually developing, physically, intellectually and emotionally: reconstructing self and environment in the process of living. 'Life-project', for Nietzsche (and commensurate with Kierkegaard and Epictetus) was a form of continuous individual self-impulsion. As appropriately summed up by Ralph Waldo Emerson:

> I make my circumstance. Let any thought or motive of mine be different from that they are, the difference will transform my condition and economy. I – this world which is called I – is the mould into which the world is poured like melted wax. The mould is invisible but the world betrays the shape of the mould.
>
> (Emerson 1981, 95)

Common to these different writers is an awareness of what might be termed 'existential power' (Rapport 2005). Individual human consciousness defines its own objectives, and projects these into and as the world. Existentially, power can be conceived of as an inherent attribute of individual embodiment whereby human beings constitute and reconstitute the meaningful environments in which they live, through their ongoing activity-in-the-world effect their own worlds. Such existential power can be conceived of as something metabolic – something pertaining to individuals as discretely embodied physical organisms – and more exactly as something intelligent, pertaining to the capacity to sense and make sense. Through willed activity-in-the-world and personal assessment of what the senses relay, individual identities develop: a personal sensorium in which consciousness dwells. A unique, individual history of environmental engagement unfolds and grows that encompasses its own ways of doing and being, its own habits and logics. 'Life-project' is a way to capture how individuals attend to and interact with what is around them, and through this attention, this interaction, form identity and environment alike. Their life-project is to be appreciated as affecting the choice of relationships, human and non-human, in which that individual engages, and the way they conduct these. Their life-project causes specific reactions to events – to a recognition of certain things in an environment as 'events' – and causes the construing of certain things as resources towards effecting personal goals. An environmental architecture emerges, a kind of personal space: a life-project amounts to a personal and subjective ecology, homeostatic conditions extending beyond the integument of the skin by which individual lives are conducted.

Individual life-projects give rise to a particular bodily hexis: to the texture of an individual life, to a specific engagement with time and space, its patience and haste, to the discipline imposed on the self, and the meanings, values, identities and relations derived from those engagements.

The life-project of personal health and wellbeing

The main argument of this chapter is that included in the recognition of an individual's life-project and the existential power that each individual possesses to direct a life are individual habits of health and wellbeing. Human consciousness, embodiment and environmental hexis form a whole that is specific to an individual life. To do justice to the nature of individuality in a system of modern healthcare is to apprehend the personalism of the environment that is an individual's habitual, healthy (homeostatic) way of being. Through their life-projects individuals maintain a set of life-conditions within which they mean to flourish in their own healthy ways, according to notions of wellbeing derived from their own histories of personal, homeostatic, engagements with the world.

As exemplification, let me adduce a narrative of Allison James's, in her article "The Standardized Child: Issues of Openness, Objectivity and Agency in Promoting Childhood Health" (2004). James's argument is that medical science has been integral to the establishing of norms in health – such as child growth and development – which, while offering beneficial measures against which human life can be judged, can also work to stigmatize individuality as pathological. The standardization of norms may operate as a kind of coercion, even tyranny, as if 'healthiness' were necessarily universal.

James elaborates. Nineteenth-century utilitarian interest in the physiology of the developing human body led to a surveying of child populations that gradually began to define certain 'objective' standards of normality for 'childish' bodies. This charting had great significance with respect to political and social policy interventions and was instrumental in improving the life-chances of otherwise marginal children (enabling patterns of growth retardation to be detected and ameliorative welfare measures to be instituted). However, what also developed has been a kind of 'surveillance medicine' ostensibly still part of a benign state regime of legislative care. No longer simply focused on the epidemiological mapping of disease and the monitoring of growth, statistics on child ill-health now entail processes of regulation and control through which children's bodies come to be coercively 'constituted' by adult carers. The hidden costs of democratically recognizing a population for an inclusive benefitting from modern medical science – drawing up of standards against which individuals can assess their health status, identifying risky behaviours, publicly disseminating knowledge – have seen individuals being identified as categories of persons, such as 'children'. Standardization and an essentializing of human identity have replaced a recognition of and respect for individuality.

The issue, James insists, is as much scientific as ethical. Standardized models of child growth and development, ideas of essential human normalcy, are a spurious veneer on actually diverse realities. 'The standard child' is a misnomer: a dangerous misrecognition of the essential variation within any actual human population. "Until medical science can be used to celebrate diversity", James urges (2004, 107), both to "widen our visions of normalcy and to permit children more participation as social actors in respect of their own health status", we risk an unethical paternalism and an unscientific essentialism. To imagine a twenty-first-century 'liberal welfarism' (Dworkin 1977) might be to commit to an inclusiveness and 'uniformity' that treat the individuality of human embodiment. Self-awareness, self-management and the assumption of health rights might be watchwords, within strategies of health promotion that recognize the extents of personal 'responsibility' for definitions of healthiness and wellbeing.

Healthcare as modern technology and cosmopolitan recognition

Fundamental to the human condition as theorized by Gregory Bateson was an appreciation of the 'cybernetic' or recursive connection between the psychological and the biological. "We commonly think of the external 'physical world' as somehow separate from an internal 'mental world'", Bateson wrote (1972, 429, 441), however it would be truer to say that "the mental world – the mind, the world of information processing – is not limited by the skin" and that there is a 'mental determinism' which is immanent in the world of all living creatures. The physiology of the human organism is thus a matter of feedback (manifested as transfers of energy) between purposive actions and evaluative reactions to their effects. A recursive processing of information causes not only ideational or imaginal effects but physical ones too.

The claim of this chapter has been that an individual's interpretation of, and intentions towards, the world – as an ongoing personal history – give rise to the phenomenon of individual-in-its-environment as a thing in itself. Caused by a lifetime of attending, in a distinctive way, to what the senses relay concerning the body's circumstance and activity, individuals come to occupy distinctive spaces which are at once cognitive, affective and physical. Through habits of environmental engagement, human beings structure distinctive, personal life-worlds that include their own versions of health and wellbeing.

Moreover, the individual-in-its-environment is something to which a liberal society may aim to do increasing justice, as scientific practice and as moral practice alike. Modern technologies add to the capacity of regimes of institutional healthcare to discern individualities of healthy embodiment: how each 'patient' occupies a life-world that is distinct and discrete. Equally, modern technologies may be made available as a form of equal opportunity: furthering innate individual capacities to engineer life-worlds that reflect an individual authorship. Finally, modern technologies have the potential to make a unified world in which opportunity is equalized on a global scale, and the patient is simply 'Anyone', any individual human being (Rapport 2012).

If life-projects are conceived of as manifestations of a human existential power to make worlds that reflect the will of their individual creators, and if these worlds are conceived of as including the physical, homeostatic conditions of healthy embodiments by which a life comes to be individually characterized, then a liberal system of healthcare might ideally hope to ensure that globally, as a cosmopolitan project, human beings should have the right to medical recognition of the specificity and the personality of their wellbeing. The environment of their healthy embodiment becomes, indeed, an individual's personal preserve, globally protected from external (cultural, social, medical) definition and appropriation.

References

Bateson, G. 1972. *Steps to an Ecology of Mind*. New York: Ballantine Books.

Dworkin, R. 1977. *Taking Rights Seriously*. London: Duckworth.

Edelman, GM. 1992. *Bright Air, Brilliant Fire: On the Matter of the Mind*. London: Penguin.

Emerson, RW. 1981. *The Portable Emerson*. Revised ed. New York: Penguin.

James, A. 2004. "The standardized child: Issues of openness, objectivity and agency in promoting childhood health." In *Democracy, Science and the 'Open Society': A European Legacy*, edited by N Rapport. Münster: LIT Verlag Münster. 93–110.

Mill, JS. 1909. "On liberty." In *John Stuart Mill: Autobiography, Essay on Liberty; Thomas Carlyle: Characteristics, Inaugural Address, Essay on Scott; with Introductions and Notes. Vol. 25, Harvard Classics*, edited by CW Eliot. New York: PF Collier & Sons.

Murdoch, I. 2001. *The Sovereignty of Good*. London: Routledge. Original edition, 1970.

Nietzsche, FW. 1968. *The Will to Power*. New York: Vintage Books.

Rapoport, A. 1998. "Spatial organization and the built environment." In *Companion Encyclopedia of Anthropology*, edited by T Ingold. New York: Routledge. 460–502.

Rapport, N. 1993. *Diverse World-Views in an English Village*. Edinburgh: Edinburgh University Press.

Rapport, N. 2005. *I am Dynamite: Alternative Anthropology of Power*. London: Routledge.

Rapport, N. 2012. *Anyone, the Cosmopolitan Subject of Anthropology*. New York: Berghahn Books.

Rapport, N. 2018. "The action and inaction of care: Care and the personal preserve." *The Australian Journal of Anthropology* 29 (2):250–257. doi: 10.1111/taja.12290.

Tallis, R. 2001. "The truth about lies: Foucault, Nietzsche and the Cretan paradox." *Times Literary Supplement*.

Turner, JS. 2000. *The Extended Organism: The Physiology of Animal-Built Structures*. London: Harvard University Press.

4 Socio-narratology and the clinical encounter between human beings

Arthur Frank

When the door of a room in a clinic or a hospital closes, what we call *healthcare* is individual people co-constructing a story. This story begins in mutual uncertainty; it may end quickly or continue to be told after one participant's death. The story is acted out in multiple encounters, each affected by what happened before and affecting what follows. The people in those rooms cannot just make the story develop any way they choose; each person's options are limited by multiple factors. But none of the participants is without choice.

Encounters between people make up only a small part of healthcare. Changing what happens in these moments will not transform the institutional, financial, political, scientific, or professional structuring of healthcare. My interest is in offering people – both ill people and professionals – resources with which they can make small but not insignificant changes that affect how they experience each other: individual people's sense of being helped or hindered, energized or drained, redeemed or rejected by each other.

Socio-narratology as narrative care

Among the activities that collect under the rubrics of health humanities, medical humanities, or healthcare humanities – each of these labels carrying different implications for who participates and who is in some way served (Frank 2019) – arguably the most concentrated attention has been devoted to narrative. Some narrative approaches involve teaching literature as a means of enhancing the interpretive and empathic capacities of clinicians to listen to their patients (Charon et al. 2016). Other approaches draw upon family therapy for innovative ideas about how to ask questions that have therapeutic value for patients (Launer 2018). These approaches support each other, but they have distinctive ways of working that reflect the different institutional situations of those whose publications elaborate each approach. Narrative approaches to health or medical humanities continue to proliferate (Stagno, Blackie, and Frank 2019).

What I call *socio-narratology* (Frank 2010) asks social scientific questions – questions about how people affiliate into groups, define the boundaries of these groups, and sustain shared interpretations of reality – using concepts drawn from literary and folklore studies of narrative. Socio-narratology overlaps with other work in health humanities, but offers a different way of thinking and practicing. Influences on socio-narratology begin with studies in folklore (Propp 1968) that show how a story is fabricated: stitched together from shared narrative resources that include character types and recognizable plot structures. Socio-narratology emphasizes the *dialogical* nature of interaction, considering how each communicative move is made in anticipation of another's response and how each act is ethical insofar as it establishes a relationship between self and other (Bakhtin 1983; Frank 2004). Third on this incomplete list of influences are social scientific studies (Latour 2005) that lead me to understand stories as *actors*. Socio-narratology studies stories *doing things*; stories act. Stories act for people; people do things with stories. Equally important but less obvious, stories act *on* people, doing things to them. For socio-narratology, stories are crucial *mediators* of what constitutes people's reality. Humans need the mediation of stories in order to make reality coherent and be able to articulate what counts as experience. The concern of this chapter is not theoretical elaboration. Instead, I seek to show how to put socio-narratology to work in clinical settings.

I describe clinical work based on socio-narratology as *narrative care;* that phrase implies both care *through* narrative means and also care *of* people's narratives. These two forms of care affect two entwined forms of storytelling: first, the *ongoing enacted narrative,* that is, the story that people are co-constructing as they encounter each other in clinical settings; second, stories that people retell to themselves and others that orient and guide them. Which stories people retell and enact depends on their *narrative habitus.*

The sociologist Pierre Bourdieu (1990) defined habitus not simply as people's habits, but as the dispositions that give rise to these habits and are reinforced by them: matters of personal taste and beyond that, a sense of what counts in life, what is worth taking seriously. *Narrative* habitus begins with a corpus of stories, many learned early in life, that people know in whole or part and retell to themselves and others. Narrative habitus expands to comprise a person's disposition as to which stories are *worth paying attention to* and which stories can be ignored; which stories are funny, scary, wise or foolish, appropriate to tell and to whom, or keep secret, and maybe dangerous. Stories have multiple dangers, only some of which people are reflectively aware of. Because stories sort out realities, they usually limit what can be perceived as possibilities. To recognize that stories guide action does not imply they necessarily guide people in directions of human flourishing. Stories justify violence as often as they create empathy – that is their danger.

The quality of *care* in narrative care is a disposition that is cultivated and reinforced through practices involving narratives. To suggest how narrative care might work in clinical settings, I propose seven areas of question-openings. These are not necessarily questions that clinicians ask patients directly. Instead, they mark areas of systematic curiosity that can be explored in questions suited to specific contexts, phrased in language appropriate to those involved. In an ideal clinical world, questioning would include clinicians asking about patients, patients being curious about clinicians, and people questioning themselves as a narrative self-analysis.

Question-openings of narrative care

These seven question-openings of narrative care are presented in an order that is iterative; that is, later questions build on earlier ones and reopen earlier discussions, adding new dimensions. This list is in *no sense complete*. The point is for people to adapt it, reshape it through experience, and use it to reflect on themselves and to practice being curious about others.

First, which stories are a person's active *companions*? Once at a fairly large conference I was on a panel discussing care. When questions were invited, a medical resident wearing green scrubs elaborated the multiple irresponsibilities of her low-income patients, ending with why these justified the clinic's disciplinary actions toward offenders. Her companion stories were about patients missing appointments, failing to take prescribed medications, and so forth. Those stories accompanied her and affected expectations that included new patients. The stories justified her practicing medicine in an attitude of generalized resentment. I sat there wondering what stories her patients told about her and how those stories, as their companions, created their expectations for future healthcare encounters.

To know someone requires knowing what stories they hold as companions, because *those stories hold them*. In my ideal clinic, clinicians meeting patients for the first time would ask about the patient's past experiences of seeing doctors and other health professionals, and then about family stories of previous illnesses and care. They would ask for stories describing when things went well and badly. Clinicians would also ask each other what their stories are, and invite reflections on how these stories are affecting their expectations and actions that make these expectations into self-fulfilling prophecies.

Second, which narrative type is the present story part of? *Stories* in my usage are about specific times and places; they describe characters marked as particular. *Narratives* are generalized types of stories. This distinction draws upon an organizing device in folklore studies, the tale type. A tale type is a recognizable plot and character structure that informs multiple specific stories. Thinking in tale types makes recognizable similarities between stories told in different cultures and in different historical periods. The titles of many of the stories collected by Jacob and Wilhelm Grimm have become tale types; the most prominent example may be Cinderella (Pullman 2012). It makes sense to describe a contemporary film or novel as a Cinderella story. In my usage, it's technically a Cinderella *narrative* that gives shape to those specific stories that follow a recognizably similar progress of events: initial oppression (perhaps after a fall from an earlier state of privilege), ordeals in this oppression, finding a helper (the fairy godmother figure), a period of preparation, a contest in which the hero is aided by resources given by the helper, and finally triumph over the oppressors. The medical resident described earlier was telling stories that followed a medically recognizable non-adherence narrative, which is a specific form of the more generally recognizable blaming narrative. Patients also tell stories recognizable as blaming narratives, but these stories blame healthcare workers, as well as employers and friends who are not supportive.

Narratives are cultural resources, but they are shared unevenly. Groups, or relationships of mutual understanding and affinity, are held together by members sharing certain preferred narratives and their complementary disuse, maybe suspicion, and possibly demonization of other narratives. People who work in clinical care prefer what I have called the *restitution* narrative (Frank 2013), in which persons get sick, receive medical treatment, and return to a good enough version of their life before illness. Patients are cued to understand what happens to them within this narrative; that is, to interpret treatment events and effects within the frame of expectations that this narrative sets in place. Medical end-of-life care also has a *futility* narrative, according to which further treatments will have no curative benefit and care should be directed only at comfort. The drama of end-of-life care involves who makes this shift between narratives, when actors shift, who sticks with restitution in some form, and what one participant must do to affect others' preference between narratives.

Placing stories in narrative types frees thinking from the specificity of stories. Stories are best at capturing the here-and-now of events, and the contingent particulars of people, places, and acts. That story work is important, but stories can hold people too close to particulars. Thinking in narratives offers distance. Narrative types reveal similarities and tensions between stories: which go well together and which are incompatible. It is more useful to ask which narratives shape the stories told in specific groups than to endlessly elaborate the multiple specific stories that are told. Also, how a specific story plays against its narrative type suggests insights into what problems the storyteller has narrating his or her life.

Third, what is the story's *narrative logic*? Narrative logic means who, in the world of the story, is able to do what, and what are the expected or possible effects of different actions – how do things turn out, for whom, doing what? Stories presuppose a narrative logic, and then reaffirm this narrative logic as a reasonable, even necessary way to understand the world. In the medical resident's blaming narrative, some people try to help other people and those other people capriciously undermine being helped. Especially when telling stories in a public setting, storytellers reaffirm their own belief that their world works this way, and they enlist listeners to share the narrative logic the story presumes. Storytelling validates the world as storytellers and their listeners know it.

Narratives tend to remain silent about why some things happen, and those silences are significant. In the resident's narrative, a significant silence is why those who undermine help are acting that way. Action is individualized, and individuals are decontextualized. Those people's backstories of what made them who they are, and their side-stories of what they now respond to, are left out. A complementary silence can be heard in patients' blaming narratives, although these generally contain phrases that gesture toward an unknown context, such as: "I know they're busy but . . .".

In healthcare, effective, efficient, and ethical practice – both the practices of clinicians and those of patients – depends on all participants sharing *sufficiently* similar narrative logics. That sharing gets more complicated as narrative logics become twisted, or can seem twisted to those who live according to different narrative logics. Patients with life threatening conditions and their families are told that treatments are effective and worth whatever dislocation and side-effects, until a moment when clinicians declare that efficacy has stopped. Relationships are further complicated when narrative logics are left implicit, as they usually are. Healthcare workers generally do not spend time asking patients and families whether they share a belief that medical treatments are generally effective; they do not solicit and explore doubts that patients might have. If patients and families have difficulty articulating their goals and doubts, that is in part because they lack listeners with whom they can practice speaking what they feel, and in part because their narrative logics are twisted by conflicting desires and wrong or partial information.

Gaining trust and cooperation requires knowing a person's narrative logic – again, beliefs about what is possible for what kinds of people to do, with what effects resulting from that doing. Thinking how stories fit into narratives enables specifying the narrative logic with which a storyteller is operating in his or her world, or recognizing twists in someone's narrative logic.

Fourth, how did the *characters* in people's stories get to be who the story presents them as being? To enact the stories people live as their lives, they *cast* others – as a theatre director casts a play – in roles the imagination of which comes from the storyteller's companion stories. Institutions are also cast in character types – for example, as helpers or antagonists. How people cast others sets expectations, and again, expectations often become self-fulfilling prophecies.

Two crucial differences emerge if we consider how different people cast those whom they encounter. One difference involves complexity, or what literary critics call *rounded* characters versus characters who are either good *or* bad, helpers *or* antagonists. Rounded characters can be helpful in some matters but then troublesome in others; they surprise us, or maybe we allow them to be surprising. Another axis of difference is between castings that reflect the storyteller's generalized expectation that the world is basically friendly, versus the expectation that the world is adversarial, exploitive and unfair. Narrative care seeks to help people reflect on where they sit on these two axes of difference. It also assists in reflecting on how you yourself are being cast in others' stories, and why those others need you to play that part.

Fifth, most stories are *communal*, and questions ask what community or communities support the continued telling of any particular story. Stories circulate and gain support within families, professional groups, friendship groups, faith communities, and leisure groups, and these groups have meeting places. In healthcare, doctor's lounges, nursing stations, lunch places, and patient support groups – many of which are now in the virtual space of the internet – are all places where people support the telling of stories that fit particular narratives. Specific questions about the communal basis of stories include asking people where they hear and tell stories, whose stories they hear and who listens to their stories, and what stories they hear other people telling about experiences like theirs. These stories help in understanding what keeps people oriented to the stories they take seriously.

The opposite aspect involves which communities a storyteller believes would not know or be able to understand her or his stories. Which communities are predictably antagonistic to which stories? At the extreme, would the storyteller feel threatened if some communities knew she or he were telling a particular story?

Sixth, how *committed* is a person to particular stories and narratives, and to specific interpretations of those? Both healthcare professional groups and patient support and advocacy groups often require a high level of members' commitment to particular narratives. This commitment tacitly or explicitly denies that its most shared stories admit multiple interpretations. Eliciting commitment to interpretive lines is a pivotal moment for groups. I once co-presented a workshop with a colleague who evoked scenes from her father's end-of-life care. He had been a farmer, and when his adult children and wife had to make decisions about whether treatment should end, they told stories about his remarkable survival of several illnesses and farm accidents that could have killed him. Those stories in themselves could have supported either a narrative that their father and husband had suffered enough and subjecting him to more medical treatment was cruel, or they could support a narrative of "Dad's a fighter" and imply continuing treatment. Family members had to commit to one line or the other. Communities circulate more than stories. Groups support interpretations of those stories and are more or less demanding about adherence to those interpretations. In both medical grand rounds and patient support groups I have seen attempted expressions of alternative ways of understanding shut down.

Seventh, what *conflicts* does a person or group's adherence to a story or narrative create with other groups? Others might reject a story on multiple grounds that include: its basis in fact, its omission of relevant aspects of what happened, false assumptions that its interpretations rest on, and the story's contradiction with principles that the conflicting group is committed to upholding. Some stories are inherently conflictual, for example, stories of past wrongs inflicted on storytellers and their groups. In many stories, conflicts start with which narrational point of view is given priority, because any narrator's point of view carries with it values and predispositions that the narrator considers unquestionable, but some listeners consider highly questionable. Healthcare professionals, patients, and patients' families are each often convinced of the rightness of their privilege in telling the version of the story that everyone else should accept and act upon. Narrative care never assumes anyone's privilege.

To return to the meaning of *narrative care*, caring for narratives involves being willing to listen to other people's stories with generosity. The relevant questions while listening are not whether the story is right or wrong, but rather what this story does for the person telling it. What needs does it fulfil? The needs a story addresses are real, even if the story is wrong, and sometimes a story needs to be wrong to fill a need. Some stories once filled a need, but they no longer do so. In my earlier example, people who are recently diagnosed may need a restitution narrative. But when curative treatment is no longer working and may be increasing the patient's discomfort, then what doctors and ethicists call a futility narrative is kinder. Although, using the word *futility* is rarely kind and may generate a narrative conflict. Doctors mean to say that further treatment is futile. Patients and family readily hear that as saying their life is futile. Narrative care takes most seriously the words that evoke different narratives.

Narrative care often proceeds by telling people stories they had not thought of as relevant, or by reminding them of stories they themselves once told but then set aside. Those stories bring new interpretive possibilities to a situation. The basic premise is that people need stories in order to make their experiences coherent and that stories are told by reassembling resources from other stories. People recreate stories from fragments of other stories, while being committed to the uniqueness of stories they call their own. Care works by offering more resources people can use to recreate stories that are better companions. What *better* means in any specific clinical context will vary with that context and be a work in progress, always evolving. Narrative care does not anticipate outcomes; on the contrary, it regards anticipations as dangerous because they inhibit flexibility to persons and events. Socio-narratology seeks to expand people's breadth and depth of curiosity and interest, not to tell people what do.

Conclusion: transforming what?

Narrative care works like water: it seeps into cracks and gradually opens these into larger spaces. If narrative care aspires to transform healthcare, it seeks to do so one story at a time. Or more specifically, narrative care works through one *relationship* at a time. That relationship is between someone telling a story that they believe does something for them and a listener who respects that need but holds open the possibility that the immediate story may not be doing what the teller needs. Listeners need to consider their own narrative predispositions: which narratives they take most seriously, what interpretations and judgments those narratives lead to, and which narratives they are predisposed to dismiss. We all do things with stories. And we all live among stories that are doing things to us.

References

Bakhtin, M. 1983. *The Dialogic Imagination*. Austin: University of Texas Press.

Bourdieu, P. 1990. *The Logic of Practice*. Translated by R Nice. Stanford: Stanford University Press.

Charon, R, S DasGupta, N Hermann, ER Marcus, and M Spiegel. 2016. *The Principles and Practice of Narrative Medicine*. New York: Oxford University Press.

Frank, AW. 2004. *The Renewal of Generosity: Illness, Medicine, and How to Live*. Chicago: University of Chicago Press.

Frank, AW. 2010. *Letting Stories Breathe: A Socio-Narratology*. Chicago: University of Chicago Press.

Frank, AW. 2013. *The Wounded Storyteller: Body, Illness, and Ethics*. 2nd ed. Chicago: University of Chicago Press.

Frank, AW. 2019. "The voices that accompany me." *Journal of Medical Humanities* 41 (2):171–178.

Latour, B. 2005. *Reassembling the Social: An Introduction to Actor-Network Theory*. New York: Oxford University Press.

Launer, J. 2018. *Narrative-Based Practice in Health and Social Care: Conversations Inviting Change*. London: Routledge.

Propp, V. 1968. *Morphology of the Folktale*. 2nd ed. Austin: University of Texas Press.

Pullman, P. 2012. *Grimm Tales: For Young and Old*. London: Penguin.

Stagno, S, M Blackie, and AW Frank. 2019. *From Reading to Healing: Teaching Medical Professionalism Through Literature*. Kent: Kent State University Press.

5 Interrupted body projects and the narrative reconstruction of self

Andrew C Sparkes

If, as Shilling (2013) suggests, the body is a changing resource and an unfinished project that individuals work on, and invest in, throughout their lifespan, then it is a precarious project that can be interrupted at any time due to, for example, traumatic spinal cord injury (SCI). Interrupted body projects like this bring about dramatic change in the material body and the social and psychological worlds that people inhabit. In such circumstances, the tendency is for people to turn to narrative (Medved and Brockmeier 2008; Sparkes 2015). They do so because these bodily changes have meaning, and narrative is the language of meaning. Within this process, as Frank (2013) points out, the body speaks, and corporeal character of the body as an obdurate fact shapes the kind of stories that come out of it and how they are received and understood. Thus, Heavey (2015) talks of *narrative embodiedness*, a central aspect of which is the ever present material, fleshy, *object body* as the *source* and *topic* of a narrator's stories that shape not only *what* can be told about subjective experience but also *how* it is told to self and others.

The object body is not free to construct just any story it wishes about itself. Although the corporeal experiences and the reported biographical events may be unique to the individual, as Gubrium and Holstein (2009) remind us, the narrating subject is enmeshed in a social world, and no item of experience is meaningful in its own right but is made so in the narrative work and practices that people actively engage with in a social context. Within this interactional terrain, people assemble their stories by "artfully picking and choosing from what is experientially available to articulate inner lives and social worlds" (2009, 30). Regarding this artful selection, McAdams (2006) and Medved and Brockmeier (2008) suggest that culture provides people with a limited menu of narrative forms and contents that contain a broad repertoire of genres, plots, models, and storylines from which they can selectively draw to make sense of, and give meaning to, their interrupted body projects.

With regard to the cultural menu on offer, people are drawn to some stories over others due to their narrative habitus that is shaped via complex processes of socialization associated with, for example, social class, gender, ethnicity, religion, ableness, sexuality, and so on. According to Frank (2010) a narrative habitus involves the gradual embedding of stories in bodies in ways that predispose people to hear some stories as those that they ought to listen to, ought to repeat, and ought to be guided by because they *feel* that some stories are *for* them, or not for them, by expressing possibilities of which they are or can be part, or by representing a world in which they have no stake.

The problem

People who experience a SCI that results in permanent disability can encounter a range of physical and psychosocial health-related complications. These complications can be alleviated by engagement in leisure-time physical activity (LTPA), defined as physical activity an individual engages in during their free time such as playing sport, or exercising in the park or a gym (Martin Ginis et al. 2010). Despite this, most people with SCI live insufficiently active lifestyles with an estimated 50% being completely sedentary (Smith, Perrier, and Martin 2016).

Post-SCI narratives and their influence on LTPA: examples of restitution and quest

Given the issues raised in the introduction, and the sedentary lifestyles associated with SCI, it is important to better understand how different narratives made available to people post-SCI shape the ways in which they experience their object body and influence their decisions to engage in LTPA. In what follows, therefore, I consider the influence of two specific narrative types, that of restitution and quest (for other types see Frank 2013; Smith and Sparkes 2008, 2011).

A life history study of a group of men who suffered a SCI and became disabled due to playing rugby union football, revealed how during their rehabilitation in specialist units, and on their return to the community, the dominant narrative on offer to them to reconstruct their body-self was that of *restitution* (Smith and Sparkes 2002; Sparkes and Smith 2002, 2008, 2011). This work also illustrated how the narrative habitus of these men, informed by a strong athletic identity and the disciplined bodies they had developed through sporting practices and training regimes prior to SCI attracted and predisposed them to notions of restitution.

The restitution narrative, according to Frank (2013), has the following plot line: "Yesterday I was healthy, today I'm sick, but tomorrow I'll be healthy again" (2013, 77). For the men in the study by Sparkes and Smith (2002) whose sense of masculinity had been influenced by their socialization into sport, this translated to, "Yesterday I was able-bodied, today I'm disabled, but tomorrow I'll be able-bodied again". Within this narrative, certain metaphors (Smith and Sparkes 2004), time tenses (Sparkes and Smith 2003), and kinds of hope (Smith and Sparkes 2005) worked in combination to give meaning to the past, current, and future bodies inhabited by the men. For example, within the restitution narrative, sporting or 'war' metaphors were prominent. The most common was associated with a *fight* to make a *comeback* and closely linked to the belief that biomedicine would be able to find a 'cure' for SCI. These men also spoke of *winning* as being *cured* of disability that is an *enemy* that must be *beaten*. Such metaphors connected to how autobiographical time in this narrative was experienced within a philosophy of the future, such as the tense of *future in the past* (in the future I will be able-bodied again just like I was in the past). Here, stories are told to the self and others of a future that is predicated on gaining a *restored* self via medical advances so that the body's former predictability is regained. In turn, this led to a *concrete* sense of hope that is oriented to specific or material results and realizing desirable outcomes (e.g., walking again).

Having lived within the restitution narrative for a number of years it is interesting to note that several of the men in the study by Sparkes and Smith became dissatisfied with it because it was not working for them and gradually gravitated towards a *quest* narrative which allowed them to experience and inhabit their bodies in very different ways (Frank 2013). This narrative meets suffering head on, accepts disability, and seeks to use it in the belief that something is to be gained from the experience. Within this narrative, very different metaphors, time tenses, and senses of hope were in operation. For example, the most prevalent metaphors used by these men were that of the *journey* and being *reborn*.

The quest narrative is associated with a *fragmentary* model of autobiographical time that recognizes the unpredictable nature of human life and the complexity of self which leads to different tenses being used from that of the restitution narrative (Brockmeier 2000). For example, the *future being in the past* tense of restitution is replaced by the tense of the *future in the future* (what the future holds is uncertain and cannot be predicted). This leads to the possibility of *transcendent* hope that embraces uncertainty and finitude, celebrating surprise, play, novelty, mystery, and openness to change. Here, the hopeful person, rather than being defined or enslaved by a particular outcome, is continually open to the possibility that life will disclose as yet unknown sources of meaning and value. In quest, therefore, becoming disabled through sport is reframed as a challenge and an opening to other ways of being in the world that allow a *developing* self to emerge. By opting for such a self, these men emphasized their ability to reconstruct their sense of embodiment over time, they displayed an openness to change, and they showed a willingness to explore new identities and bodily experiences as possibilities emerge.

Given their characteristics, the restitution and quest narratives offer different possibilities for people post-SCI to make sense of their interrupted body project and the reconstruction of self. For example, in terms of people with SCI being involved in LTPA, the restitution narrative may motivate individuals for instrumental reasons to engage in LTPA because they want to maximize their chances of gaining a restored self of self via a cure for paralysis. In contrast, those people living post-SCI within the quest narrative are likely to engage in LTPA in a more intrinsic and open manner as part of a developing self that is willing to explore new identities and experiences via their object body as it currently is and could be in the future.

A number of studies that have focused on LTPA post-SCI support the views expressed earlier. For example, in their life history study of Dan, a professional wheelchair bodybuilder, Sparkes, Brighton and Inckle (2018a) illustrate close links to Dan's previous sense of self with a strong athletic identity as a committed amateur bodybuilder pre-SCI and his decision to engage in this activity, only far more seriously and successfully, post-SCI. In part, Dan's decision was framed by his narrative habitus that drew him to the restitution narrative following his interrupted body project that then led him to seek a hyper-muscular restored self. Likewise, drawing on an ethnographic study conducted by Brighton (2014) of why people who have become disabled due to SCI choose to engage with, and experience, wheelchair sports post-SCI, Sparkes, Brighton and Inckle (2018b) suggested that, for the participants in this study, the athletic identity they developed pre-SCI, coupled with the influence of the restitution narrative, played an important role in them engaging in wheelchair sport post-SCI. Significantly, over time, through prolonged and intense practice they became highly skilled users of their wheelchairs, incorporating it into their body and seeing it as an extension of their self in the process of what Papadimitriou (2008) describes as becoming *en-wheeled*. As part of this process, these athletes constructed and took pride in their new identity and their re-embodiment as a disabled sporting cyborg that directly challenged ableist views of disabled people as tragic, weak, powerless, and passive.

A direct link between the restitution narrative and people with acquired disability engaging in LTPA is made in the study by Papathomas, Williams, and Smith (2015) when they speak of *exercise is restitution* as a narrative type that, driven by a desire to move again and restore the body to its former, pre-injured state, people are motivated to keep training and continue their exercise regimes. This narrative emphasizes LTPA as a means to a 'cure' for SCI where the teller is reliant on future medical discoveries to maintain a sense of concrete hope.

Finally, in their consideration of narratives of athletic identity after acquiring a permanent physical disability, the *athlete as a future self* as described by Perrier et al. (2014) has traces of restitution within it. This is because those using the narrative type of *athlete as a future self* still made constant comparisons between past and present selves. Significantly, however, the point of comparison for this group is behaviour as opposed to changes to the physical body and its performance capabilities, and this enabled them to keep their future identity as athlete open. These participants felt, therefore, that although their present behaviour was not in line with that of an athlete (as they were), an athletic identity could be restored once their future behaviour changed as they participated in a new sport or returned to the same sport, provided that it could be adapted to their needs.

The restitution narrative in various guises can, therefore, motivate some people, particularly if their narrative habitus draws them towards it and they have developed a strong athletic identity, to engage in LTPA post-SCI. This narrative type can, however, be problematic (Frank 2013; Sparkes and Smith 2011). For example, if the person did not have an athletic identity or engage in LTPA pre-SCI then any restored self that is constructed post-SCI is unlikely to rush out and take up LTPA. Even if a strong athletic identity had been developed pre-SCI, the perceived gap between the physical function and performance capabilities of the pre- and post-SCI body may be deemed too great and impossible to restore. This, as Perrier et al. (2014) point out, leads to the development of a *nonathlete narrative* in which any possibility of approximating a restored self is defined as 'mission impossible' and this can deter people from engaging in any LTPA.

In addition, for some, the ideology of ableism plays a role in their decision to become involved in sport post-SCI. For example, Sparkes and Smith (2002) indicated that several of the men in their study who adhered to the restitution narrative would not entertain any involvement in wheelchair sport as they defined this as 'crip' sport for the disabled, that is the 'other' not 'them'(Smith and Sparkes 2004). Finally, there is the deep rooted problem identified by Papathomas, Williams, and Smith (2015) that if the motivation to engage in LTPA is predominately inspired by the goal of recovery and a fully restored self, as opposed to a goal of enjoyment, social interaction, or developing a new sense of body-self and trying out different identities, then what happens when functional restoration plateaus and full recovery is not forthcoming? One answer is that the person becomes demotivated and withdraws from LTPA. As Papathomas et al. point out, given the permanency of paralysis caused by SCI, the notion of 'waiting for a cure' represents a troubling predicament for those holding the *exercise is restitution* narrative. For them, this predicament can lead to psychological disruption that occurs when one's personal experience is misaligned with one's personal story and is unlikely to facilitate continued LTPA engagement.

Another response to the predicament described earlier, as evidenced in the work of Sparkes and Smith (2002, 2003, 2011) and Smith and Sparkes (2004, 2005), is the gradual recognition by people post-SCI that the restitution narrative is not working for them and that it may in fact be acting in their lives as what Craib (2000) calls a narrative of *bad faith*. Such narratives, he suggests can be restrictive, functioning to keep people in passive positions, inhibit possible change, and separate people from the authenticity of their lives. Such recognition initiates movement away from restitution and towards the quest narrative that, given its characteristics described earlier in relation to SCI, opens up different possibilities for engagement in LTPA.

Signs of the quest narrative opening up different possibilities post-SCI for engaging in LTPA are evident in the *present self as an athlete* narrative described by Perrier et al. (2014) that is informed by the philosophy of "I act, therefore I am". People in this group focused predominantly on their present behaviour, though past performance and future goals were also identified as heavily influential on athletic identity. Importantly, however, this comparison involves the immediate past and near future, and does not involve direct comparisons between the pre- and post-SCI selves. Rather, in the present self as athlete narrative, the pre- and post-SCI selves are seen as different people. Here, for the current self, present behaviour and future goals in sport are of central importance as is a commitment to training, practicing, and participating in competitions as this allows for identification with the athletic role as an evolving process. All of this can be accomplished without the need to compare and measure oneself with the body-self pre-SCI with a view to restoration, allowing greater freedom for a developing self to regularly engage in various sports and LTPA.

The influence of the quest narrative is also present in the *exercise is progressive redemption* narrative type identified by Papathomas, Williams, and Smith (2015). The plot line of this progressive narrative is characterized by an upward trajectory of overcoming challenges towards some positive outcome of self-improvement or personal betterment. Here, according to McAdams et al. (2001), the process involves a transformation from a bad, affectively negative life scene (e.g., SCI and paralysis) to a subsequent good, affectively positive life scene in which the bad is redeemed, salvaged, mitigated, or made better in light of the ensuing good (e.g., becoming involved post-SCI in STPA again or for the first time). As Papathomas et al. point out, this narrative fuels a desire to try for progression and improvement along with a commitment to succeed in the face of adversity which is a useful commodity when pursuing an active lifestyle post-SCI. Papathomas et al. suggest that subscribing to this narrative may facilitate resilience against the many barriers to LTPA that people with SCI face and that, therefore, it represents a potentially useful narrative resource for the promotion of LTPA in the SCI population. For Papathomas and colleagues, the progressive redemption narrative is principally characterized by positive identity change rather than a cure from SCI and leads to a more transcendent form of hope.

Implications for practice or theory

Each narrative type mentioned earlier influences, in different ways, the motivations of people post-SCI to engage in LTPA. For those living their lives post-SCI and those supporting them it is important that they are provided with opportunities to become aware of the narrative type they are drawing on and what draws them to this type in the first place. They can then consider whether this narrative is working for or against them in both the short and long-term. For example, whilst notions of restitution may be useful early on post-SCI and during rehabilitation in specialist units, it may become increasingly less useful and more constraining as time goes on. Here, narratives influenced by notions of quest might become more appropriate. In such circumstances, people post-SCI need to be made aware that other narrative types exist and be given the opportunity to reflect on what the adoption of different narratives might mean for them in their lives. Given the power of the narrative habitus any attempt at narrative transformation is difficult and will require timely, informed, and strategic interventions and sustained support from relevant health professionals, family members, and friends if the person post-SCI is to engage in LTPA throughout their life span.

Conclusion

In terms of SCI as an interrupted body project, and the decisions of people post-SCI to engage in LTPA, narratives of various types play a crucial role in this decision-making process which can have long-term consequences for their health and wellbeing. Therefore, to support people who encounter a major interrupted body project of any kind we need to better understand what narratives are made available to them and how these perform, work, and act in their lives. Such an understanding will allow health practitioners and others to assist people post-SCI in the process of narrative transformation if, and when, the opportunity arises, so that they can choose those narratives that enable them to become the body-selves they seek in the future and enhance their various ways of being in the world.

References

Brighton, J. 2014. "Narratives of spinal cord injury and the sporting body: An ethnographic study." PhD, Leeds Beckett University.

Brockmeier, J. 2000. "Autobiographical time." *Narrative Inquiry* 10 (1):51–73.

Craib, I. 2000. "Narratives in bad faith." In *Lines of Narrative: Psychosocial Perspectives*, edited by M Andrews, S Sclater, C Squire, and A Treacher. London: Routledge.

Frank, AW. 2010. *Letting Stories Breathe: A Socio-Narratology*. Chicago: University of Chicago Press.

Frank, AW. 2013. *The Wounded Storyteller: Body, Illness, and Ethics*. 2nd ed. Chicago: University of Chicago Press.

Gubrium, JF, and JA Holstein. 2009. *Analyzing Narrative Reality*. London: Sage.

Heavey, E. 2015. "Narrative bodies, embodied narratives." *The Handbook of Narrative Analysis*:429–445.

Martin Ginis, KA, AE Latimer, KP Arbour-Nicitopoulos, AC Buchholz, SR Bray, BC Craven, . . . PJ Potter. 2010. "Leisure time physical activity in a population-based sample of people with spinal cord injury part I: Demographic and injury-related correlates." *Archives of Physical Medicine and Rehabilitation* 91 (5):722–728.

McAdams, DP. 2006. "The role of narrative in personality psychology today." *Narrative Inquiry* 16 (1):11–18.

McAdams, DP, J Reynolds, M Lewis, AH Patten, and PJ Bowman. 2001. "When bad things turn good and good things turn bad: Sequences of redemption and contamination in life narrative and their relation to psychosocial adaptation in midlife adults and in students." *Personality and Social Psychology Bulletin* 27 (4):474–485.

Medved, MI, and J Brockmeier. 2008. "Continuity amid chaos: Neurotrauma, loss of memory, and sense of self." *Qualitative Health Research* 18 (4):469–479.

Papadimitriou, C. 2008. "Becoming en-wheeled: The situated accomplishment of re-embodiment as a wheelchair user after spinal cord injury." *Disability & Society* 23 (7):691–704.

Papathomas, A, TL Williams, and B Smith. 2015. "Understanding physical activity participation in spinal cord injured populations: Three narrative types for consideration." *International Journal of Qualitative Studies on Health and Well-being* 10 (1):27295.

Perrier, M-J, SM Strachan, B Smith, and AE Latimer-Cheung. 2014. "Narratives of athletic identity after acquiring a permanent physical disability." *Adapted Physical Activity Quarterly* 31 (2):106–124.

Shilling, C. 2013. *The Body and Social Theory*. London: Sage.

Smith, B, M-J Perrier, and JJ Martin. 2016. "A partial overview and some thoughts about the future." *Routledge International Handbook of Sport Psychology*:296.

Smith, B, and AC Sparkes. 2002. "Men, sport, spinal cord injury and the construction of coherence: Narrative practice in action." *Qualitative Research* 2 (2):143–171.

Smith, B, and AC Sparkes. 2004. "Men, sport, and spinal cord injury: An analysis of metaphors and narrative types." *Disability & Society* 19 (6):613–626.

Smith, B, and AC Sparkes. 2005. "Men, sport, spinal cord injury, and narratives of hope." *Social Science & Medicine* 61 (5):1095–1105.

Smith, B, and AC Sparkes. 2008. "Changing bodies, changing narratives and the consequences of tellability: A case study of becoming disabled through sport." *Sociology of Health & Illness* 30 (2):217–236.

Smith, B, and AC Sparkes. 2011. "Exploring multiple responses to a chaos narrative." *Health* 15 (1):38–53.

Sparkes, AC. 2015. "When bodies need stories: Dialogical narrative analysis in action." In *Advances in Biographical Methods*, edited by M O'Neill, B Roberts, and A Sparkes. London: Routledge. 50–62.

Sparkes, AC, J Brighton, and K Inckle. 2018a. "Imperfect perfection and wheelchair bodybuilding: Challenging ableism or reproducing normalcy?" *Sociology* 52 (6):1307–1323.

Sparkes, AC, J Brighton, and K Inckle. 2018b. "'It's a part of me': An ethnographic exploration of becoming a disabled sporting cyborg following spinal cord injury." *Qualitative Research in Sport, Exercise and Health* 10 (2):151–166.

Sparkes, AC, and B Smith. 2002. "Sport, spinal cord injury, embodied masculinities, and the dilemmas of narrative identity." *Men and Masculinities* 4 (3):258–285.

Sparkes, AC, and B Smith. 2003. "Men, sport, spinal cord injury and narrative time." *Qualitative Research* 3 (3):295–320.

Sparkes, AC, and B Smith. 2008. "Men, spinal cord injury, memories and the narrative performance of pain." *Disability & Society* 23 (7):679–690.

Sparkes, AC, and B Smith. 2011. "Inhabiting different bodies over time: Narrative and pedagogical challenges." *Sport, Education and Society* 16 (3):357–370.

6 The *Fourth Research Paradigm*

Activating researchers for real world need

Frances Rapport and Jeffrey Braithwaite

Revisiting the qualitative-quantitative debate

In medical and health services research we have for too long been locked into an unresolved debate about the merits of qualitative research – that apparent 'poor cousin' to quantitative research when it comes to generating robust evidence. The debate, which still rumbles on, includes arguments about: 1) the degree to which qualitative data should be considered data in its own right, 2) whether qualitative data is as impactful as quantitative data, and 3) whether qualitative data isn't at its most useful as either a pre-cursor to quantitative data or as a way of evaluating quantitative data (Piil et al. 2013; Lakshman et al. 2000; Rapport, Bierbaum et al. 2018). This debate often concludes with qualitative data being under-valued; seen only in terms of its complementarity to quantitative data; a mere accompaniment to quantitative questions, hypotheses or numerical findings; or as an unreliable or non-generalizable accoutrement.

The debate extends, however, into an examination of qualitative methods' main qualities. People hold strong views that qualitative data are 'soft' data, dependent on researcher flexibility, personal position-taking (unhelpfully also known as personal bias or personal prejudice) and a subjective lens (Noble and Smith 2015). These qualities, so the argument goes, are unlike those of quantitative data, with its 'hard' edges, clear structure and objective, more readily verifiable findings. The debate invariably leads to quantitative data being lauded as 'the Real McCoy'.

Consequently, different fields of thought have embraced or rejected qualitative methods, pitting them against quantitative methods which are often perceived as more rigorous, with opportunities for greater penetration into creating evidence-based outcomes. We argue here that in the future, we might wonder though why we ever bothered weighing one up against the other. As digitization grows and information transforms the world, we have a genuine opportunity to benefit from multiple data sources. By cross-referencing gold standard Randomized Controlled Trials (RCTs) with richly detailed social observations of the activities of clinicians and patients, data collected in situ alongside a constant stream of digital data can help break new ground in triangulating the who, the why and the wherefore of effective healthcare. This includes healthcare in all its permutations, including healthcare settings and systems, service development and delivery, service appraisal and policy development, and ethical and governance considerations. This would take us well beyond the unproductive quantitative versus qualitative debate, which, among other things, prompted 76 academics from 11 countries to petition the *British Medical Journal* over the privileging of quantitative studies in its pages, despite qualitative studies' higher citation rates and enviable contributions to healthcare and human health (Greenhalgh et al. 2016).

Surely, we should be harnessing the unfolding, data-rich landscapes of medicine and healthcare research more effectively than we currently do? We've been wedded to quantitative research for far too long, because of its scale and the confidence that comes from statistically robust, easy to encapsulate and digest findings. But any study predicated on summarizing its results according to a handful of numbers is, by any definition, imperfect and at the very least, lacking substance, and findings are determined, as for all research, by personal judgements about what is valuable and worthy of measurement (Krauss 2018). Even when we measure, we would point out that numbers are simply an abstraction of reality, even in the most well-cited articles, such as the 3.2% reduction in depression scores following online cognitive behavioural therapy (Christensen, Griffiths, and Jorm 2004), or the 19 in 10,000 healthy menopausal women at risk from combining oestrogen and progesterone (Writing Group for the Women's Health Initiative 2002). What do numbers such as "3.2% reduction" and "19 in 10,000 women at risk" really mean for patients?

Why we should not dismiss qualitative research out of hand

Qualitative research has often been dismissed as little more than a series of case studies. Interesting and informative, yes, when it comes to shining a spotlight on that fluid web of human interactions that make healthcare tick, but unhelpful for extrapolation and generalization to a wider cohort of patients, professionals and members of the general public. Yet qualitative studies can tell us a great deal. They can point to, for example, why clinicians do not always apply an evidence-base to their clinical judgements (because of difficulty in keeping up to date, and other barriers) (Grossman 2018). Nor do practitioners necessarily follow formal guidelines, but rather trust in their own personal judgements when it comes to treatment and care: mindlines not guidelines, in a famous paper (Gabbay and le May 2004). This is known as personal 'equipoise', the approach to decision-making which favours, despite the evidence, one's worldview: "I have always done it this way and I have no intention of changing". Equipoise has been seen to affect not only people's everyday practices, but also their perceptions of the world around them, including the value they place on professionalism, different drugs and therapeutic regimes, and decision-making skills (Williams et al. 2016).

Qualitative studies can also tell us a great deal about how people communicate, down to the smallest detail of the conversations they have, within and beyond a formal consultation context. Conversation analysis, for example, can examine the impact of a loaded pause or a rhetorical turn of phrase (Jones 2007), while discourse analysis can follow a storyline, tracing styles of speech and speech patterns through a range of conversational pathways (Elwyn and Gwyn 1999). These methods can progress our knowledge of shared decision-making, patient and professional interaction, co-created care, and many other aspects of discourse, and can help circumvent problems in meaning-making. Moreover, these kinds of studies can help clarify the integrity of professionals' day-to-day work, and the value they place on others' actions (Elwyn et al. 2012).

The *Third Research Paradigm (Mixed Methods Paradigm)*

More recently, moves to integrate quantitative and qualitative research methods have led to the *Mixed Methods* or *Third Research Paradigm* (Gunasekare 2015), such that neither quantitative nor qualitative data are privileged, but both are used together, wherever they contribute best, to support a more fuller understanding of the subject and object of enquiry. This paradigm has helped for example clarify care pathways, from primary to tertiary care, and from tertiary care back into the community, indicating how patients are empowered or isolated as they enter, remain or exit healthcare settings. These kinds of studies, which blend, mix or intermingle quantitative and qualitative data, can triangulate knowledge and illuminate how care works or where it is falling short (Dixon-Woods et al. 2014; Hutchings et al. 2016; Johnson et al. 2017; Pool et al. 2010). Such studies endorse the benefits of having complementary data and select research methods based on pragmatic notions of what data have in common, how they fit together to provide a fuller picture of the world being investigated, and their ability to coalescence around common themes or phenomena (Johnson and Onwuegbuzie 2004).

Johnson and Onwuegbuzie (2004) present the importance of the *Third Research Paradigm* according to the paradigm's pragmatic aspects. At a theoretical level they refer to its ability to: reject the traditions of dualism in favour of workable solutions to problem-solving, foreground action over philosophizing and minimize reductionist tendencies. Johnson and Onwuegbuzie (2004) list a wide range of mixed methods' characteristics, which together speak to the paradigm's practical empiricism. This recognizes that the world is ever-changing and that people are constantly adapting to new situations. The characteristics have led to a useful set of guidelines that offer researchers a steer on mixed methods in use, including how to recognize weaknesses in quantitative or qualitative data, and where combining them can strengthen understanding.

Yet, in an era where the knowledge explosion means there are 30 million publications listed in Pubmed, the electronic database of health and medical research, there are 75 randomized trials and 11 systematic reviews published every day, and the half-life of medical knowledge is as little as a few years and growing ever-shorter, we still need something more. We need a dialogue that extends beyond a refutation of quantitative method's strict objectivity, a new paradigm to move methodology forward. By introducing a paradigm shift in this chapter, we wish to take advantage of the dynamic interface between healthcare's people, places, objects, technologies, activities and time. We want to introduce methods that are flexible enough, and sensitive enough, to catch a glimpse of the messy world of healthcare professionals and care delivery, and that can record patients' fears and anxieties, dreams and aspirations, as quality of life improves or degrades. To capture this, we wish to make a case for a new set of methods which we call 'mobile methods'. These we recommend qualitative researchers add to their repertoire, so that they can go out into the world and conduct work 'on the hoof' alongside research subjects.

The *Fourth Research Paradigm*

Plans for mobile methods to become more mainstream in medical and health services research have led to our predictions for a *Fourth Research Paradigm* (see Table 6.1, Principal Features). Currently, mobile methods are very much the domain of anthropologists and sociologists (Bates and Rhys-Taylor 2017; Brown and Durrheim 2009; Kusenbach 2003). However, we are testing their qualities and opportunities through a number of feasibility studies in health, designed to accommodate a rapidly changing health service environment, with methods that are flexible and rigorous.

While the *Fourth Research Paradigm* is still in its infancy and may well expand beyond mobile methods approaches, studies undertaken in the United Kingdom and Australia are bearing fruit in revealing the complexity of health systems, and which are preludes to *Fourth Research Paradigm* studies. These include, to cite just four examples: 1) a study of the impact of university gyms across England and Wales on staff and students' health, wellbeing and organizational affiliations (Rapport, Hutchings et al. 2018); 2) the influence of gastroenterological surgical workspaces on staff identity, patient and professional safety and wellbeing (Auton et al. 2019); 3) an examination of how clinicians' pace at work helps explain their culture and efficiency (Braithwaite et al. 2018); and 4) a study of 32 hospitals

Table 6.1 The *Fourth Research Paradigm*: Principal features

Epistemology	*Fluid, Creative, Exploratory*
Data type	Mobile, Shared, Emergent
Researcher-subject relationship	Democratic, Equalizing, Adaptive
Researcher position	Partner, Listener
Methodology	Performative, Science-Social Science, Ethnographic, Poetic Representation
Methods	Multiple methods from other paradigms, plus Technological Data (Smartphones, Apps), Social Media Data, Performance, Biographies and Photographs, Everyday Objects, Obscure Phenomena, Auto-biography
Data characteristics	Nuanced, Ambiguous, Complex, Anomalous, Flexible

Source: Adapted from Rapport, F, and J Braithwaite. 2018. "Are we on the cusp of a fourth research paradigm? Predicting the future for a new approach to methods-use in medical and health services research." *BMC Medical Research Methodology* 18 (1):131.

and how they are organized to deliver quality care, and the extent to which they achieve that goal in practice (Taylor et al. 2015).

These studies reveal the messy, habituated practices that are taking place every day, across large and small organizations (such as universities and hospitals), and their effect on organizational development. The studies also indicate how people make accommodations to suit one another or their environment, cleverly adapting not only themselves but also their setting to fit in better.

Research activity in the *Fourth Research Paradigm*

The *Fourth Research Paradigm*'s mobile methods' activities centre around the necessity for researchers and participants to come together, to reflect on a variety of issues relating to specific research questions, and as they do so, to move (temporarily on an equal footing) through time and space. They will share qualitative, quantitative and mixed methods data, and discuss them, and they will do so in real time.

One mechanism under the banner of the *Fourth Research Paradigm* is to conduct discussions as researchers and participants walk and talk together. Whether formal or informal, recorded or noted, for a few minutes or over lengthy periods, this can reveal insights and clarity of detail that is rarely achieved through static data-capture. Mobile methods also appear to stimulate a greater thoughtfulness in people's comments, and a degree of openness rarely evident in interviews or focus groups (Boase and Humphreys 2018). In effect, 'walking and talking' within a setting where people work, live or spend their leisure time, acts to stimulate 'trigger points' (see the following section) to truthful exposition.

Walking and talking also allows memories to surface, while movement can help to contextualize deeply held views about situations and settings, as they unfold in front of the researchers and participants, leading to more pertinent conversations. This can also lead to others joining in. And so, reflections open up to other conversations.

Walking and talking is invariably a sensory experience, revealing a person's emotional investment in people, places and in themselves. Movement across and within the settings where research conversations are being held can indicate the degree to which healthcare practices and personal perspectives are embedded in everyday function: Why do I want to go to the gym? Do I want to feel part of a treatment group? Is the data suggesting I am getting well? How engaged am I in my treatment compared with others?

Trigger points

Trigger points, stimulated by mobile methods, are 'eureka moments' when a new thought occurs, something important is said or done, or an impactful event is experienced. Trigger points can be derived from something the research participant, the researcher or others say or do. Others are those people external to, yet somehow part of, the research event, such as patients, family, friends, students, gym buddies, managers, technicians or healthcare professionals. But others can also be people with nothing to do with the original encounter, who are not linked to the research group, but share the same public or private domain.

When a trigger point occurs, one or more of the people involved can choose what to do about it, whether to make it apparent and pursue it further, and whether to record it or move beyond it to the next trigger point. For the researcher, this includes whether to address the moment or take the experience further, while the research participant can choose how to describe and define the moment, if at all, and what they wish to share with the researcher or others, as a result. While this may not be done knowingly, researchers are often able to pick up on these moments, applying the information to their research evaluation.

The 'work' of keeping mobile methods relevant, active and ongoing demands considerable effort on the part of the researcher. Frequently, for example, trigger points lead to relationships of greater complicity and complexity. And while they can offer a rare opportunity to share precious moments with someone else, they can also lead to queries that cannot simply be answered by a 'yes' or a 'no'. Furthermore, using mobile methods, it is possible to uncover extensive personal details about someone, stimulated by the sights and sounds that they encounter, and the researcher will have to think on their feet about how to handle this.

Others, also implicated in the mobile methods activity for a greater or lesser period of time, including colleagues, peers, friends, loved ones, outsiders, staff, students and the general public, to name but a few, become the subject or the object of the activity. In this respect, while the mobile methods approach is inclusive, it can herald complex data and scenarios that need careful management, while researchers should recognize that chance encounters can generate unpredictable events.

Researchers should consider whether the intimacy and unpredictability of this suits their and their research participants' needs, and whether these methods will bring greater quality to their data or a greater burden. And they should reflect on whether the relationships they form and the pathways they travel will enhance or restrain further contact and commitment. In effect, researchers must recognize that mobile methods can present a very different side to qualitative research than that with which they are familiar, leaving them with observations and visual or textual data that could be considered 'too hot to handle'.

A second mechanism in the *Fourth Research Paradigm* is digitally enabled mobile methods. The patient here can access as much information as they need, typically via handheld devices, apps and wearables. Details synthesized from test results, treatment progress and medical notes are provided in forms suitable for patients' needs, and feedback about changes in vital signs, information about adherence to medication and the like, is made available in a constant stream as the patient makes his or her way in life. The mobile patient is constantly in touch with progress and is fed back information in real time through text messages, Skype consultations, emails, web access, phone conversations and many forms of social media.

If researchers are prepared to take a leap of faith, mobile methods can offer rich insights into the world of people's health and healthcare delivery and enable positive feedback loops in support of patients and their progress. Although we named the *Fourth Research Paradigm* (Rapport and Braithwaite 2018) as a new phase in health and medical research, it occurs to us that it is the culmination of a maturing of and extrapolation of existing progress in health and medical research once we arrived at a good understanding of the benefits of mixed methods research, and a digitally enabled health system began to emerge. As it unfolds, the *Fourth Research Paradigm* will initiate a further wave of research; as a constant stream of data that is fresher, more flexible and more realistic than that derived from a controlled trial, or experimental study, becomes the norm. Mobile methods are destined to uncover new insights into people's behaviours that are, as of yet, undocumented. This includes: the accommodation of people and places across space and time, the circumvention of problems (also known as 'work arounds'), challenges to healthcare provision at the coal-face of care delivery, and the enabling of self-correcting health delivery systems and patient responses to the information they receive. Recognizing how the tracing of activities and interactions can affect a new wave of embodied knowledge signals a radical change to our thinking around health and illness.

Active knowing

In essence, the *Fourth Research Paradigm* introduces a new dimension to research, one of *active knowing and responding in dynamic environments*. We think the *Fourth Research Paradigm* will lead to a new understanding of those private and public healthcare services that people depend upon and it will bolster the potential for new lifestyle choices and improved health status. Patients will have all the data they need by which to make informed choices. By shadowing and supporting people in person or digitally, and by accessing their unique insights into their ecosystems, health and desires, we have opportunities to build a real world understanding of the relationships being played out in the messy universe of the healthcare provider and the patient.

This will demand much from the research community. Investigators will have to venture out of their disciplinary bunkers more often, to handle a fluid stream of data. But all stakeholders stand to be richly rewarded with a unique appreciation of the complex world of healthcare provision as it unfolds, captured as systems react and people meet, greet, interact and react.

By integrating this flow of information with freshly minted qualitative and quantitative studies, via technology, observations and informal conversations, we could generate research findings that are contemporary and relevant. Quite simply, we will know much more about how patients respond, progress or decline, and how health systems contribute to these responses, progressions or declines. If we can also build continuous feedback loops from the public to providers, and providers back to the public, perhaps we can create a 'learning system' for all, in stark contrast to today's static, clunky, hierarchical and outmoded 'forgetting system'.

References

Auton, E, R Clay-Williams, J Cartmill, J Braithwaite, and F Rapport. 2019. *Final Report: Fit for Purpose? Organisational Productivity and Workforce Wellbeing in Workspaces in Hospital (Flourish): A Pilot Study.* Sydney, Australia: Australian Institute of Health Innovation.

Bates, C, and A Rhys-Taylor. 2017. *Walking Through Social Research.* New York: Routledge.

Boase, J, and L Humphreys. 2018. "Mobile methods: Explorations, innovations, and reflections." *Mobile Media & Communications* 6 (2):153–162.

Braithwaite, J, LA Ellis, K Churruca, and JC Long. 2018. "The goldilocks effect: The rhythms and pace of hospital life." *BMC Health Services Research* 18 (1):529. doi: 10.1186/s12913-018-3350-0.

Brown, L, and K Durrheim. 2009. "Different kinds of knowing: Generating qualitative data through mobile interviewing." *Qualitative Inquiry* 15 (5):911–930.

Christensen, H, KM Griffiths, and AF Jorm. 2004. "Delivering interventions for depression by using the internet: Randomised controlled trial." *BMJ* 328 (7434):265.

Dixon-Woods, M, R Baker, K Charles, J Dawson, G Jerzembek, G Martin, . . . P Ozieranski. 2014. "Culture and behaviour in the English national health service: Overview of lessons from a large multimethod study." *BMJ Quality & Safety* 23 (2):106–115.

Elwyn, G, D Frosch, R Thomson, N Joseph-Williams, A Lloyd, P Kinnersley, . . . S Rollnick. 2012. "Shared decision making: A model for clinical practice." *Journal of General Internal Medicine* 27 (10):1361–1367.

Elwyn, G, and R Gwyn. 1999. "Stories we hear and stories we tell: Analysing talk in clinical practice." *BMJ* 318 (7177):186–188.

Gabbay, J, and A le May. 2004. "Evidence based guidelines or collectively constructed "mindlines?" Ethnographic study of knowledge management in primary care." *BMJ* 329 (7473):1013.

Greenhalgh, T, E Annandale, R Ashcroft, J Barlow, N Black, A Bleakley, . . . S Ziebland. 2016. "An open letter to the BMJ editors on qualitative research." *BMJ* 352:i563.

Grossman, DC. 2018. "Quality of health care for children: The need for a firm foundation of trustworthy evidence." *JAMA* 319 (11):1096–1097.

Gunasekare, ULTP. 2015. "Mixed research method as the third research paradigm: A literature review." *International Journal of Science and Research (IJSR)* 4 (8).

Hutchings, HA, K Thorne, GS Jerzembek, WY Cheung, D Cohen, D Durai, . . . IT Russell. 2016. "Successful development and testing of a method for aggregating the reporting of interventions in complex studies (Matrics)." *Journal of Clinical Epidemiology* 69:193–198. doi: 10.1016/j.jclinepi.2015.08.006.

Johnson, M, R O'Hara, E Hirst, A Weyman, J Turner, S Mason, . . . AN Siriwardena. 2017. "Multiple triangulation and collaborative research using qualitative methods to explore decision making in pre-hospital emergency care." *BMC Medical Research Methodology* 17 (1):11.

Johnson, RB, and AJ Onwuegbuzie. 2004. "Mixed methods research: A research paradigm whose time has come." *Educational Researcher* 33 (7):14–26.

Jones, A. 2007. "Admitting hospital patients: A qualitative study of an everyday nursing task." *Nursing Inquiry* 14 (3):212–223.

Krauss, A. 2018. "Why all randomised controlled trials produce biased results." *Annals of Medicine* 50 (4):312–322.

Kusenbach, M. 2003. "Street phenomenology: The go-along as ethnographic research tool." *Ethnography* 4 (3):455–485. doi: 10.1177/146613810343007.

Lakshman, M, L Sinha, M Biswas, M Charles, and NK Arora. 2000. "Quantitative Vs qualitative research methods." *Indian Journal of Pediatrics* 67 (5):369–377.

Noble, H, and J Smith. 2015. "Issues of validity and reliability in qualitative research." *Evidence-Based Nursing* 18 (2):34–35.

Piil, K, M Jarden, J Jakobsen, KB Christensen, and M Juhler. 2013. "A longitudinal, qualitative and quantitative exploration of daily life and need for rehabilitation among patients with high-grade gliomas and their caregivers." *BMJ Open* 3 (7):e003183.

Pool, R, CM Montgomery, NS Morar, O Mweemba, A Ssali, M Gafos, . . . A Nunn. 2010. "A mixed methods and triangulation model for increasing the accuracy of adherence and sexual behaviour data: The microbicides development programme." *PloS One* 5 (7):e11600.

Rapport, F, M Bierbaum, C McMahon, A Lau, S Hughes, and I Boisvert. 2018. *Final Report: Behavioural and Attitudinal Responses to Cochlear Implantation in Australia and the UK.* Sydney, Australia: Australian Institute of Health Innovation.

Rapport, F, and J Braithwaite. 2018. "Are we on the cusp of a fourth research paradigm? Predicting the future for a new approach to methods-use in medical and health services research." *BMC Medical Research Methodology* 18 (1):131. doi: 10.1186/s12874-018-0597-4.

Rapport, F, H Hutchings, MA Doel, B Wells, C Clement, S Mellalieu, . . . AC Sparkes. 2018. "How are university gyms used by staff and students? A mixed-method study exploring gym use, motivation, and communication in three UK gyms." *Societies* 8 (1):1–16. doi: 10.3390/soc8010015.

Taylor, N, R Clay-Williams, E Hogden, V Pye, Z Li, O Groene, . . . J Braithwaite. 2015. "Deepening our understanding of quality in Australia (Duqua): A study protocol for a nationwide, multilevel analysis of relationships between hospital quality management systems and patient factors." *BMJ Open* 5 (12):e010349. doi: 10.1136/bmjopen-2015–010349.

Williams, JG, MF Alam, L Alrubaiy, C Clement, D Cohen, M Grey, . . . A Watkins. 2016. "Comparison of infliximab and ciclosporin in steroid resistant ulcerative colitis." *Health Technology Assessment* 20 (44):1–322. doi: 10.3310/hta20440.

Writing Group for the Women's Health Initiative, I. 2002. "Risks and benefits of estrogen plus progestin in healthy postmenopausal women: Principal results from the women's health initiative randomized controlled trial." *JAMA* 288 (3):321–333.

Part 2

Systems

Part 2, Systems, is the middle section of the volume. It is a departure from the theoretical and philosophical aspects of qualitative methodological development, taking some of the 'Ideas' presented in Part 1 and examining their relationship to healthcare systems' developments. In Part 2 the systems that surround the healthcare service such as the management of operating theatres and good management's ability to build greater resilience into healthcare teams through simple reorganisation (Mahmoud et al., Chapter 8), the use of resources such as drugs and their dispensing system (Saurin and Ferreira, Chapter 7), the examination of Work-As-Imagined and Work-As-Done on hospital wards (Clay-Williams et al., Chapter 9), patient journeys through care, using patients' longitudinal healthcare experience data in novel narrative formats (Lamprell et al., Chapter 10), working hours and work patterns and insights from doctors' writings about burnout and stress (Lamprell et al., Chapter 11), and systems for treating chronic conditions like epilepsy and the consequent implications for patient disease-management (Shih et al., Chapter 12) are all examined through a qualitative lens.

Across the pages of Part 2, authors concentrate on macro, meso and micro levels of care, paying particular attention to aspects indicated in system-delivery, while considering processes and mechanisms that allow care to be provided well; such as groups of professionals working together, and less well; such as individual healthcare practitioners working in isolation. Part 2 describes both smooth and fractured pathways through care, but in each case using qualitative methods to highlight attempts to transform systems into more efficient, high-quality and safe settings for patients, using transformative and insightful methods. Part 2 also presents some of the key notions for change: the importance of improving use of 'slack resources' (such as extra people, finances or devices in space), the value of teamworking and group cohesion, the need to understand exactly how work is done and what people's routines are to reduce variability, the value of 'whole story' investigations of health and illness that include the patient perspective; but the need also to explore the doctor's experience through novel narrative writings, in order to respect the values and accomplishments that doctors have regarding the patients they treat, and the importance of sharing decisions with patients as a step forward in managing barriers to optimal communication for clearer system function. Part 2 links 'Ideas' in Part 1 to solutions to systemic problems in the health service, having taken the reader through a journey into the wider context of healthcare systems on a global scale. Through an examination of healthcare systems in Australia, the United Kingdom, the United States *of America, South America and Japan, the book raises some critical questions about whether health systems globally are failing us. By so doing, Part 2 illuminates not only system strengths, but also system weaknesses and vulnerabilities.*

The qualitative methods described in Part 2 include: observations, interviews, dialogic analyses, storytelling and narratives, online ethnography, Functional Resonance Analysis Method (FRAM), and discussions and consultation groups. In each case, methods are both exposed and dissected, so that their qualities and strengths for these kinds of investigations can be critiqued. This is supported by the presentation of a variety of case studies so the reader can follow the authors' reasoning and the researchers' decision trails.

7 Slack resources in healthcare systems

Waste or resilience?

Tarcisio A Saurin and Dayane M C Ferreira

Introduction

Healthcare is considered a complex socio-technical system due to its inherent uncertainty, diversity, and dynamics, which imply a high threshold of inevitable variability. In turn, variability can be defined as the range of values or outcomes (e.g., a patient's length of stay) around the average, as well as all possible results of a given outcome (Story 2010). Variability in healthcare is part of healthcare professionals' everyday work, since functions conducted by humans and to a degree by the technological artefacts at their disposal, tend to vary along multiple performance dimensions, such as precision and timing (Hollnagel, Braithwaite, and Wears 2013). For example, medications may not be administered at the exact prescribed dosage and time on every occasion, or may be administered differently by different healthcare professionals with the same patients on different occasions.

A common approach to the management of healthcare variability – adopted from other industries – involves attempts to enforce standardization. This approach has led to the introduction of regulatory procedures, checklists, and safety audits in several healthcare sub-systems such as surgery, clinical rounds, and intensive care units (for example, Jennings and Mitchell 2017; Ten Have et al. 2013). Notwithstanding the positive outcomes of such measures (for example, Guwande 2010), there is empirical evidence to indicate a gap remains between desired outcomes and those that are actually achieved in the workplace (Braithwaite, Wears, and Hollnagel 2016). This gap may be wider when standardization development is based on a superficial understanding of workplace realities. For example, Standard Operating Procedures (SOPs) in emergency departments (EDs) often fail to take into account the effects of overcrowding and workflow interruptions (Moskop et al. 2009).

Slack resources (used interchangeably with 'slack' in this chapter) should be considered an integral element in the design of flexible and realistic standards (Fireman, Saurin, and Formoso 2018), and more broadly as a fundamental requirement of healthcare systems. Slack, which ensures that spare resources (such as time, space, supplies, money, and staff) are available in times of need (Nohria and Gulati 1996), can cope with some of the negative aspects of variability (Safayeni and Purdy 1991). For example, slack resources can absorb the effects of variability or slow down its propagation (Perrow 1984). An example of the role played by slack resources can be found in the existence of professionals on standby in EDs. While these professionals cope with sudden surges in the demand for care (i.e., absorb the effects of variability), the ED as a whole prevents the quick propagation of variability to other hospital units. As such, slack resources can also support system resilience, which is the ability of the healthcare system to adjust its performance (for example, reallocate resources in the face of a surge in demand) prior to, during, or following changes and disturbances (such as variability), so that it can sustain a required level of performance, under both expected and unexpected conditions (Hollnagel, Braithwaite, and Wears 2013, xxv).

However, maintaining slack resources implies a cost (which may be financial, as in the cost of maintaining healthcare professionals on standby), which creates the problem of balancing the cost of slack against the benefits of slack. Too much slack can equate to waste, which corresponds with the use of more costs than can reasonably be accepted to produce a desired outcome (Shingo 1989). Furthermore, slack resources affect other elements of healthcare systems, which can give rise to unintended consequences. In complex systems these interactions cannot be fully controlled, and to some extent they develop from the self-organization of individuals and teams (Perrow 1984). A possible consequence of the emergent nature of slack resources is that over time, they may be randomly distributed across the system, and thus not match the sources of variability (Saurin and Werle 2017). In this situation, it could be said that slack resources have a downside, which we would frame as 'slack as a source of waste', as opposed to the more common view of 'slack as a source of resilience'. In this chapter, the dual nature of slack is examined via two case studies detailing the preparation and administration of drugs (PAD) in two Brazilian hospitals. Suggestions for reducing waste and enhancing resilience are also made, where appropriate.

Case studies

The two case studies were carried out in hospitals located in Porto Alegre, Southern Brazil. Case study 1 was situated in a public teaching hospital with 850 beds and 5,000 employees. It was part of a broader study in a surgical ward of that hospital, focused on improving the safety and efficiency of the PAD (Ferreira and Saurin 2019). Case study 2 was in a private hospital with 350 beds and 2,000 employees. In both cases, data collection and analysis, of the nature and use of slack resources, predominantly relied on qualitative data from interviews, documents, and participant and non-participant observations (Table 7.1).

Study 1: Slack as waste

In examining automated dispensing cabinet (ADC) utilization, the collected data indicated that the demand for the drugs stored in the ward's two ADCs peaked between 7:00am and 7:59am, since 8:00am was the standard time for administering patient medications in the morning. Because changes of shift between

Table 7.1 Overview of the case studies

	Study 1: public hospital	Study 2: private hospital
Aims of the study	This study aimed to understand the reasons for the unlevelled demand of drugs stored in two automated dispensing cabinets (ADCs)[1] in a surgical ward. There were queues to retrieve drugs from the ADCs in certain times, while they were idle most of the day. The queues delayed the administration of drugs. Based on this, the ultimate intention of the study was to level the demand and therefore improve the efficiency of the ADCs.	This study aimed to identify safety vulnerabilities in the process of dispensation of drugs in the hospital's central pharmacy, which supplied drugs to all units.
Relevance of the study for the analysis of slack resources	There were two identical ADCs located side-by-side in the same room in the nursing station. Both ADCs stored the same supplies. The initial hypothesis of the study was that one of the ADCs could be removed provided the demand for drugs was levelled. An underlying assumption of this hypothesis was that the additional ADC was a slack resource, because it was only necessary when demand for drugs was highly concentrated in a short period of time. This manifestation of slack could be framed as duplication of functions, which occurs when two different resources perform the same function (Clarke 2005).	There was a standardized window of time for requesting drugs from the pharmacy. However, orders out of this window could be accepted if tagged as urgent – in this case, the drugs should be dispensed in less than 20 minutes. The possibility of requesting drugs out of the standardized window of time was a form of control slack, which is defined by Schulman (1993) as individual degrees of freedom in organizational activity, with some range of individual action unconstrained by formal structures of command. However, according to data collected by the hospital management, that slack resource was overused by physicians, who used to tag orders as urgent even if they were not.
Data sources	Semi-structured interviews with four employees of the pharmacy (4 hours in total), 10 hours of direct observation, and analysis of the Standardized Operating Procedures for drugs preparation, dispensation, and administration. The interviews focused on understanding the use of the ADCs and its role in the broader process of preparation and administration of drugs.	Semi-structured interviews with four employees of the pharmacy (4 hours in total), 10 hours of direct observation, and analysis of the Standardized Operating Procedures of drug dispensation. The interviews focused on understanding how the processes in the pharmacy were affected by the urgent orders.
Data analysis	Content analysis of interview transcripts, notes from observations, and documents. Excerpts of text associated with the role played by slack resources, either as sources of resilience or waste, were highlighted by the researchers.	

1 ADCs are computerized, point-of-use management systems, which are used for both drugs and supplies, designed to improve the accuracy of pharmacy inventory and billing, streamline the distribution process, and aid in securing narcotics (Paparella 2006).

healthcare professionals occurred from 7:00am to 7:15am, the available time for the whole process of preparation and administration of drugs (PAD) was about 45 minutes. Other than during this peak period each day, the ADCs were not significantly in demand. As such, the use of slack resources (in this case, the second ADC) could be framed as waste during most of the day, even though it was useful during the peak of demand under the existing conditions. Indeed, the second ADC was only required for a short period due to the unlevelled demand of drugs over the day, which was assumed by management as a solvable problem. According to an interview with the ward nurse manager, the decision to use two ADCs was not based on data and facts, but rather on a conservative and intuitive approach for estimating the need for resources.

Study 1: Slack as resilience

In the course of our study of the surgical ward's use of the ADCs, two non-prescribed and therefore freely available diluents – which jointly made up 23% of demanded substances – were removed from the cabinets. The administration times of two medications that corresponded to 15% of the daily demand of medications were also moved from 8:00am to other times in the day in order to be synchronized with other medications and to level out the demand, thus reducing the number of patient visits required. It therefore became possible to transfer one of the ADCs to a unit that lacked this equipment. The relocation of this ADC made it feasible for the receiving unit to maintain a significant stock of supplies as well as to electronically track the dispensation of drugs, contributing to the enhanced resilience of the ward.

However, Ferreira and Saurin (2019) reported some problems connected with the transfer. At the original unit, the ADC was programmed to allow the dispensation of only one saline type for each patient (the reason for this was not clear). When a patient was prescribed two or more types, these were retrieved on behalf of another patient. This workaround was tolerated since all patients at the unit were covered by public healthcare insurance, and therefore patients were not individually billed. However, at the receiving unit, all patients had private health insurance, and thus a precise match between the invoice and the real consumption of supplies was required. Consequently, every time a nurse technician attempted to retrieve two or more saline types for the same patient, the ADC activated an alarm and stopped functioning. In these situations, a maintenance team was called on to repair the ADC, which was a process that could take more than an hour. This delayed the administration of drugs and could leave nurse technicians idle while awaiting the repair. Thus, this case study also illustrated the way that slack simultaneously contributed to both resilience and waste.

Study 2: Slack as waste

In this second case study, examining the use of PAD in the private hospital pharmacy, it was discovered that the urgent ordering of drugs occurred frequently – in almost 40% of cases – rather than as a last resort. Frequent urgent requests for drugs had a negative impact on patient safety, as follows:

- Urgent medications were dispensed and delivered by the pharmacy without checking for prescription errors. Instead, this check was normally made only before the second dose of the medication was given to a patient.
- Frequent, urgent requests for drugs meant that the staff involved in the dispensation of medications were often required to interrupt their work, thus increasing the likelihood of error and delaying the delivery of regular requests for drugs.

Considering this context, the physicians' degree of freedom to place urgent orders at any time played a role in waste, which in this situation implied putting patient safety at risk and reducing the productivity of the pharmacy staff.

Study 2: Slack as resilience

While the capacity of the hospital pharmacy to provide urgent medication was not a drawback in and of itself, and was necessary to enhance resilience, further investigation is needed into why this slack resource has been exploited to the point of creating patient safety hazards and efficiency losses. It is likely that the physicians who were overusing the slack resource were not fully aware of the unintended consequences of their actions. Furthermore, the interviewed pharmacy employees reported that hospital managers could be afraid of challenging practices adopted by physicians, such as the intentional mislabelling of orders as if they were urgent. The interviewees associated the management tolerance of similar practices by physicians to the fear of losing patients to other hospitals, since physicians in principle could choose to care for their patients elsewhere.

Discussion and conclusion

This chapter has explored the dual nature of slack resources in healthcare, as resilience and waste. A simplistic approach, from the perspective of the users of slack resources, would be to make more and more slack resources available. However, as demonstrated by the case studies outlined in this chapter, a slack resource may be a source of waste. In fact, given the dynamics of healthcare, the balance between slack as a source of resilience and slack as source of waste may lean more to one side than the other, depending on the context. In study 1, for example, this dynamic was illustrated by the role played by the extra ADC, which moved from an initial situation where the ADC masked waste, to a situation where it supported resilience. In study 2, the opposite dynamic seemed to have occurred. This perception is based on the assumption that the policy of placing urgent orders at any time was reasonable, before later being overused to the point of becoming a source of waste.

This changing, fluid dynamic can best be managed if information about demand and the availability of key resources to cope with demand – whether or not these are formally regarded as slack or not – is made visible in real time to all relevant agents. The said visibility can support the quick analysis of the capacity to cope with demand, underpinning decision-making on whether or not existing resources should be used, as well as the need for calling on additional resources. Misalignment between capacity and demand is a common source of undesired performance in healthcare (Anderson et al. 2016). The dissemination of information technology (IT) in healthcare (Kumari et al. 2018), such as dashboards which display information about demand (for example, pending orders for dispensing drugs, or the number of patients waiting to be seen by a clinician), and resources such as staff on duty, supplies of drugs, and numbers of available beds, can provide such information for the real time management of achieving a balance between capacity and demand.

The implications of these proposals are far-reaching, offering opportunities for further health services research. For example, the real time visibility of data related to demand and resources may affect the dynamics of social interactions between caregivers and between patients. In principle, this visibility can reduce interruptions to information exchange while at the same time it can support team decision-making based on data rather than intuition. On the other hand, visibility can make healthcare professionals more vulnerable to coercive controls and production pressures, since the mismatch between capacity and demand can be quickly identified by management.

In this respect, it would be worth taking the ideas broached in this chapter forward to an investigation of the influence of power imbalances and the broader organizational context (for example, safety culture and financial incentives for professionals) on the definition of what counts as necessary slack. This will help expand the debate on the extent to which the mismatch between capacity and demand is tolerable.

References

Anderson, JE, AJ Ross, J Back, M Duncan, P Snell, K Walsh, and P Jaye. 2016. "Implementing resilience engineering for healthcare quality improvement using the CARE model: A feasibility study protocol." *Pilot and Feasibility Studies* 2 (1):61.

Braithwaite, J, RL Wears, and E Hollnagel. 2016. *Resilient Health Care: Reconciling Work-as-Imagined and Work-as-Done*. Vol. 3. Boca Raton: CRC Press.

Clarke, DM. 2005. "Human redundancy in complex, hazardous systems: A theoretical framework." *Safety Science* 43 (9):655–677.

Ferreira, DC, and TA Saurin. 2019. "A complexity theory perspective of kaizen: A study in healthcare." *Production Planning & Control*:1–17.

Fireman, MCT, TA Saurin, and CT Formoso. 2018. "The role of slack in standardized work in construction: An exploratory study." 26th Annual Conference of the International. Group for Lean Construction (IGLC), Chennai, India.

Guwande, A. 2010. *The Checklist Manifesto*. New York: Picadur.

Hollnagel, E, J Braithwaite, and RL Wears. 2013. *Resilient Health Care*. Farnham: Ashgate Publishing, Ltd.

Jennings, FL, and M Mitchell. 2017. "Intensive care nurses' perceptions of inter specialty trauma nursing rounds to improve trauma patient care – A quality improvement project." *Intensive and Critical Care Nursing* 40:35–43.

Kumari, A, S Tanwar, S Tyagi, and N Kumar. 2018. "Fog computing for healthcare 4.0 environment: Opportunities and challenges." *Computers & Electrical Engineering* 72:1–13.

Moskop, JC, DP Sklar, JM Geiderman, RM Schears, and KJ Bookman. 2009. "Emergency department crowding, part 1 – concept, causes, and moral consequences." *Annals of Emergency Medicine* 53 (5):605–611.

Nohria, N, and R Gulati. 1996. "Is slack good or bad for innovation?" *Academy of Management Journal* 39 (5):1245–1264.

Paparella, S. 2006. "Automated medication dispensing systems: Not error free." *Journal of Emergency Nursing* 32 (1):71–74.

Perrow, C. 1984. *Normal Accidents: Living with High Risk Technologies*. Princeton: Princeton University Press.

Safayeni, F, and L Purdy. 1991. "A behavioral case study of just-in-time implementation." *Journal of Operations Management* 10 (2):213–228.

Saurin, TA, and NJB Werle. 2017. "A framework for the analysis of slack in socio-technical systems." *Reliability Engineering & System Safety* 167:439–451.

Schulman, PR. 1993. "The negotiated order of organizational reliability." *Administration & Society* 25 (3):353–372.

Shingo, S. 1989. *A Study of the Toyota Production System: From an Industrial Engineering Viewpoint*. Translated by AP Dillon. Cambridge, MA: Productivity Press.

Story, P. 2010. *Dynamic Capacity Management for Healthcare: Advanced Methods and Tools for Optimization*. Boca Raton: Taylor & Francis.

Ten Have, ECM, M Hagedoorn, ND Holman, RE Nap, R Sanderman, and JE Tulleken. 2013. "Assessing the quality of interdisciplinary rounds in the intensive care unit." *Journal of Critical Care* 28 (4):476–482.

8 Using qualitative methods to understand resilience in complex systems

Zeyad Mahmoud, Kate Churruca, Louise A Ellis, Robyn Clay-Williams and Jeffrey Braithwaite

Healthcare and operating theatres as a complex adaptive system

> We had a procedure where they were implanting a valve laparoscopically, so the surgeon is concentrating on deploying the valve and putting it in the right place and he is relying on the radiographer to say, you are in the right spot and you can deploy. But there was a lot of noise and miscommunication happened which led to the surgeon deploying it in the wrong spot and the patient passed away. Normally in an operating theatre, you have a surgeon and his assistant, an anaesthetist and his assistant, two scrub/scout [nurses] and an anaesthetic nurse. You will have around eight people maximum. But since this was a relatively new procedure for us in the hospital, we had two surgical teams, two anaesthetic teams, two sets of scrub nurses, two sets of scout nurses and a lot of technicians. So, there would have been closer to fifteen people in the room. The issue with that was that there wasn't fifteen people in the room focusing on the patient, some people were in the room waiting for their turn to do their job or were just there as stand by. So, there was a lot of background noise and chatter and what was said was that when the surgeon went to deploy the valve, there was too much noise and he misheard what the radiographer told him which made him deploy in the wrong spot.
>
> [Operating Theatre Manager]

This extract is from a qualitative research project (ongoing PhD) which we describe in greater detail later in this chapter. For now, we would like to focus on the fact that it illustrates some of the core features of healthcare delivery, including that it is: unpredictable, comprised of large numbers of different stakeholders with potentially competing priorities, dynamic, complex and sometimes even chaotic. Indeed, healthcare is increasingly recognized as a *complex adaptive system* (Braithwaite et al. 2017), meaning that its behaviour is much more like a living system than a mechanical one. It is more an ecosystem, than a machine.

Complex adaptive systems (CASs) are characterized by large numbers of diverse component parts – 'agents' (in human CASs) – that are connected to one another in a variety of ways, both directly and indirectly. Over time, the localized interactions among agents (in CASs this is termed *self-organization*) give rise to broader system level behaviours (known as *emergence*). For example, returning to our extract, we can see how the emergence of this very poor outcome (the death of a patient) was less a product of any one person's behaviour, and more the result of how the actions and interactions of the many people in the operating theatre (OT) influenced one another.

Complex systems can be understood at multiple scales (McDaniel Jr and Driebe 2001); in healthcare, we can think about the clinical microsystem, with agents such as surgeons, nurses and the patient. But we can also think about agents at a mesosystem level, in the different parts of a hospital: the clinical teams, the OT, the emergency department and intensive care unit, all interacting and affecting one another and the overall behaviour – and performance – of the hospital. At a macro level, the practices within a hospital are influenced by what is happening in political and economic arenas, and internationally too, such as, for example, in advances in new technology and procedures. Agents at this level are meta-agents and include professional bodies, government agencies, insurers, nongovernment organizations, the media and taxpayers.

Dynamic interaction between systems at multiple scales of time and space, where the rate of system change can be different for each scale, has been well studied in ecology and is termed panarchy (Allen et al. 2014). Because complex systems occur at multiple scales, conceptually drawing any boundary around 'a system' is to some extent an arbitrary decision, one that empirically sharpens our focus on particular types of agents and their interactions. However, it is important to recognize that boundaries are usually porous; agents within a system may influence and be influenced by those outside that system or by external practices, policies or directives.

Studying resilience in complex systems

Thinking about systems, and particularly complex systems, one of the key behaviours we want to understand and measure is resilience, which can be broadly defined as the capacity of a system to maintain performance in response to expected and unexpected conditions (Braithwaite, Wears, and Hollnagel 2015). In healthcare, resilient performance is often understood with reference to safety; a resilience approach to safety views humans, with their capacity to adapt to varying conditions, as a positive resource for maintaining performance, rather than the more conventional view of humans as a liability to be controlled and managed (Hollnagel and Woods 2006).

Studies of resilient healthcare have proliferated over the last half-decade (Braithwaite, Wears, and Hollnagel 2016; Hollnagel, Braithwaite, and Wears 2013; Wears, Hollnagel, and Braithwaite 2015; Hollnagel, Braithwaite, and Wears 2019), and the vast majority of these have utilized qualitative or mixed methods. Qualitative methods, particularly those that focus on sustained and in-depth deployment of a researcher in a healthcare setting, are highly amenable to studying resilience because of the dynamic and ephemeral nature of this phenomenon. Resilience is understood as something a system *does*, rather than something a system *has*; we can often only identify that a system has behaved resiliently in hindsight, so instead we look to study the system's capacity for resilience. Hence, we observe resilience as it is expressed, and unfolds, and in terms of past expressions, but even then, recognizing it is difficult (in maintaining performance, outcomes are within the 'normal' range, and therefore often inconspicuous). We are much better at noticing when things go wrong in healthcare and acting after an event has happened (Hollnagel, Braithwaite, and Wears 2013).

Furthering the study of resilience, Hollnagel developed the Resilience Assessment Grid (RAG) to assess a system's potential for resilience (Hollnagel 2010, 2011). The RAG denotes four key abilities: respond, monitor, learn and anticipate. Each of these four abilities is described in greater detail in Box 8.1, but it is important to recognize that they are, to a large extent, interdependent (that is to say, responding requires monitoring).

Box 8.1   Resilience Assessment Grid

- The ability to *respond* involves knowing what to do and when to do it. That means adapting behaviour in the face of regular changes and unexpected disturbances in a manner that is both timely and effective.
- The ability to *monitor* requires knowing what to look for both in one's own performance as well as the environment. Monitoring means paying attention to the right things, looking for cues to changes that could affect a system's performance.
- The ability to *learn* involves memory and reflection, that is, the capacity to learn from experience. It is a necessary prerequisite for improving performance. In particular, this means learning the *right* lessons from the *right* experiences.
- The ability to *anticipate* essentially means knowing what to expect. Going beyond a fairly narrow risk assessment approach, this involves recognizing the potential for future disruptions, novel demands or environmental constraints that could affect the system's capacity to operate.

The RAG can be employed in a very structured, mixed methods way, to measure a system's capacity for resilient performance. However, it can also be used, as it is in this chapter, as a framework for data analysis, in a study attempting to understand resilience (see also Zhuravsky 2019).

Case study presentation and methods

For the remainder of the chapter, we draw on data collected for a PhD research project exploring the use of industrial production models in OTs. Our case study, initiated by the quote at the beginning of this chapter, and presented later in this chapter, provides an illustration of how the RAG can be used as a framework through which to qualitatively explore resilience in healthcare settings.

Case studies are a form of empirical research used to examine phenomena when they cannot be detached from their context (Yin 2009). This research design is therefore particularly useful when trying to understand contextually embedded system characteristics such as resilience.

Hospital X is a tertiary public hospital located on the eastern coast of Australia. Founded in the nineteenth century, the hospital has a total capacity of 600 beds and is recognized as a major trauma centre providing general and specialized care in most medical and surgical specialties. Within the hospital, a state-of-the-art OT houses 18 operating rooms (ORs) used for both elective and emergency procedures. OTs are a critical area in which poor behaviour can quickly escalate and lead to devastating consequences, and this makes them a suitable field for the study of resilience. Additionally, in terms of a CAS, OTs, as a field of study, provide greater control over their boundaries than other areas of the hospital. The teams are fixed for the duration of the surgery, the time over which they work together is bounded by the beginning and end of the operation, and team functioning is bounded by the surgical space.

Non-participant observation, interviews and documentary analysis were the main data collection methods used to conduct this study. Data collection was conducted by the first author. These methods were chosen as they give primacy to the actors (also known as 'subjects' or 'research participants') and their interactions (Groleau 2003). While our data collection approach allowed the collection of rich and contextualized data, we were aware of the various subjectivities inherent in our approach and resulting from our active involvement in the data generation and collection process (Wacheux 1996). We used a data collection matrix to systematize the way we conducted our observations. Following Groleau's recommendations, the matrix was organized into three distinct columns: the first was to describe events as they unfolded during the observation sessions, including information about our location, time of day and the roles of observed participants. The second column labelled 'methodological notes' allowed us to keep track of questions that we had or certain elements that we wanted to clarify with participants. The third column was devoted to 'analysis notes'; it grouped together theoretical elements that certain events evoked and constituted a first attempt at theorizing and analyzing our data. The generic nature of the matrix allowed us to grasp a wide range of observed phenomena without overly constraining them. In total, 120 hours of observation were conducted throughout this study over a period of five weeks.

In addition to observation, we used semi-structured interviews to allow research participants to express themselves as freely as possible and discuss their work and what seemed important to them (Demers 2003). We started interviewing OT nurses after saturation of themes was reached from the observational data, that is to say, when we observed that no new information emerged during data collection activity (Morse 1995). This also enabled us to integrate some of the questions that emerged from our observations into the interview schedule. All interviews were transcribed as soon as possible after their completion.

Twenty-eight research participant interviews took place. Interviewees were selected using a purposive sampling approach to ensure a wide range of different OT staff professional groups and coverage, both at the micro- and meso-levels of the OT staff groups (Figure 8.1). The aim of the sampling strategy was to ensure that all staff groups and manager levels working in the OT would be represented in the study. This culminated in 33 hours of interview audio recordings.

To complement these two methods, we conducted an in-depth analysis of two macro-level documents: "The operating theatre efficiency guidelines" published by the New South Wales (NSW) Agency for Clinical Innovation and the NSW Auditor-General's report entitled "Managing operating theatre efficiency for elective surgery" (NSW Agency for Clinical Innovation 2014; New South Wales Auditor-General 2013). These documents offered important insights into what is expected from the OT in terms of organization, performance, training and staffing. They are an integral part of the overall context of the hospital's OT remit and were thus valuable in informing our analysis in terms of how they are used, and the extent to which they can influence resilient performance of individuals and of the OT.

Data were analyzed using a theory-driven deductive thematic analysis approach following Braun and Clark's six-step process (Braun and Clarke 2006). We started by familiarizing ourselves with the data, listening to all the interviews and transcribing them verbatim. We then proceeded to generating initial codes to synthesize and organize data. Once completed, codes were then classified into the four dimensions of resilience defined in Hollnagel's RAG (that is to say, responding,

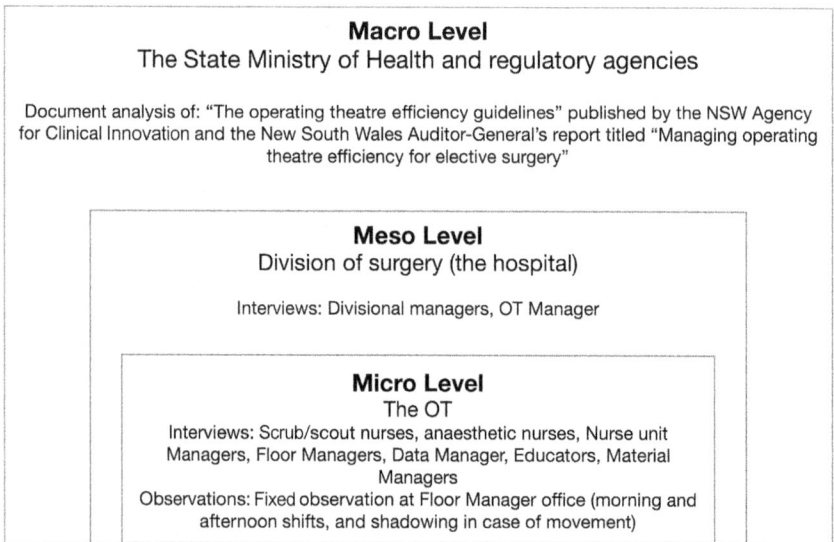

Macro Level
The State Ministry of Health and regulatory agencies

Document analysis of: "The operating theatre efficiency guidelines" published by the NSW Agency for Clinical Innovation and the New South Wales Auditor-General's report titled "Managing operating theatre efficiency for elective surgery"

Meso Level
Division of surgery (the hospital)

Interviews: Divisional managers, OT Manager

Micro Level
The OT
Interviews: Scrub/scout nurses, anaesthetic nurses, Nurse unit Managers, Floor Managers, Data Manager, Educators, Material Managers
Observations: Fixed observation at Floor Manager office (morning and afternoon shifts, and shadowing in case of movement)

Figure 8.1 Details of data collection sample.

Source: Authors' own work.

monitoring, learning and anticipating). After this, a review phase ensured the accuracy of results leading to the findings reported in this chapter.

Responding, monitoring, learning and anticipating: resilience in practice in the OT

The situation recounted in the quotation at the beginning of this chapter occurred early in this study and illustrates an example of when the OR system did not exhibit resilient behaviour. As mandated by regulation for serious incidents in Australian hospitals, the hospital conducted a Root Cause Analysis (RCA) to identify the reasons leading to the death of the patient. The goal of RCA is to draw generalizable lessons and introduce safeguards into day-to-day practice to avoid the reoccurrence of this kind of undesirable event.

Two contributing factors were found by the RCA team to have led to this event: first, an unnecessarily large number of clinical personnel present in the OR at the time the event occurred who belonged to different teams and were unfamiliar with one another. Second, noise (including chatter) in the OR which made it difficult for the surgeon to hear the radiographer, and which led him to deploy the valve in the patient's aorta. Both of these factors were not particularly unusual in the hospital, or indeed any modern hospital. In fact, during observations, we witnessed many bystanders in ORs who were either external (medical representatives) or internal (students or staff interested in learning a specific procedure). Noise was also common; indeed, some procedures we observed were conducted while music was playing in the room and it was not unusual for team members to chat as they went about their tasks. As an external observer, such distractions seemed potentially risky, but for these research participants it was just 'business as usual', demonstrating a propensity for staff to adapt and work together through variable and challenging conditions.

Nevertheless, mandatory safety 'huddles' were introduced as a direct result of the RCA by the hospital's division of surgery. The concept of a team 'huddle' (Glymph et al. 2015; Cracknell et al. 2016) was created for the TeamSTEPPS program (Alonso et al. 2006; Sheppard, Williams, and Klein 2013), to fill a role in healthcare that the 'brief' (the formalized, structured communication between team members prior to a task that has safety implications) usually fills in the aviation field. The 'huddle' is based on the idea that talking about what is about to happen, together with the opportunity for questions, creates a common understanding amongst team members and reduces the likelihood of error. It is shorter than a handover, and is usually used to communicate about specific safety risks associated with a situation, patient or group of patients (Glymph et al. 2015; Cracknell et al. 2016).

TeamSTEPPS is a healthcare team training program based on aviation Crew Resource Management teamwork training developed in the United States (US) in the mid-2000s by the US Department of Defence Patient Safety Program in collaboration with the US Agency for Healthcare Research and Quality. The implementation of this initiative was the first time we had been able to ascertain that a critical incident had recently occurred in the OT. For example, during observations, we encountered numerous posters on the walls of the theatre encouraging staff to do huddles and explaining what form they should take. These observed signs prompted new lines of inquiry during interviews about what the huddles aimed to achieve and how they had come about. In the following sections, we briefly present how the huddles supported resilience by enhancing the OT nurses' ability to learn, monitor, anticipate and respond to adverse events.

The introduction of huddles in the case study OT

Huddles were introduced at the start of each day within every OR in the hospital in question. The goal of the huddle was to increase staff's capacity to anticipate, prepare or undertake any necessary measure to avoid the occurrence of undesirable events. They started with team introductions, providing an opportunity for staff to introduce themselves and communicate their name and role for the day. Huddles were initiated by a member of the nursing team and were often led by the most senior operating surgeon, who was widely regarded as knowing the most about the patients on the list. During the huddle, case details were reviewed for each patient. These details included the patient name, the planned procedure and its estimated duration. A surgical plan was discussed, covering any specific patient requirements or potential difficulty and contingency plans for any possible adverse event. The anaesthetist discussed the type of anaesthetic that would be used and highlighted any risks, issues or concerns from an anaesthetic perspective. Nurses were responsible for communicating a nursing plan, confirming that equipment was available and accounted for, and specifying who would be carrying out the 'scrubbing up' (preparing for theatre and involved in the surgical procedure and thus remaining in the OR). The nursing plan also included communication around scouting roles (that is to say, who would be providing support during the surgical procedure, while scout nurses are also free to move throughout the OT for each procedure). Huddles and their benefits were best explained by one of the scrub/scout nurses interviewed:

> [The huddle] is inclusive and involves everyone who is involved in the patient care. So, the operational assistants, the anaesthetists, the surgeon, physiotherapist and whoever. We go through the list and talk about the operational requirements for the list. Any out of the ordinary patient indicators, any allergies, medical or comorbidity issues. That allows us to look at our whole day, plan and be proactive rather than reactive. [. . .] It gives everyone the opportunity to ask questions and clarify anything that they might not be sure about at the beginning of the day. [. . .] I think it allows us to be as prepared as possible at the start of the day. Rather than having to act in the moment.
>
> [Scrub/Scout Nurse 1]

Learning, anticipating, monitoring and responding are core aims of huddles. By sharing information about the patient and their expectations for the surgery, not only are the surgical teams engaging in communication, but they are also learning from each other. In fact, as explained by one of the nurses during an interview, the surgeons and anaesthetists often share advice with the nursing staff on how to respond in the case of an adverse event:

> From the huddle I will [. . .] ask a little bit more questions to the surgeon about what kind of things might be required if [the laparoscopy] was to go open, or what retraction does he think he will want to use, how big the incision is going to be, is it a midline incision or another kind of incision. All these kinds of things are important so that we can prep and be ready.
>
> [Scrub/Scout Nurse 2]

By sharing their expectations of how the surgical procedure should unfold, surgeons and anaesthetists also helped nurses identify the baseline 'normal state' for every procedure. This enabled them to be actively involved in monitoring the progress of the surgeries and quickly identifying anything out of the ordinary. This also greatly improved their capacity to anticipate and prepare responses to adverse events.

> It also makes us work much more efficiently and effectively as a team as well because we are able to kind of get a bit of insight on what is going on with the patient and we are able not only to bounce ideas off the surgeons or ask any queries. We are also able to kind of think for ourselves and get stuff that we can see that they are probably going to be required, maybe have them set up just outside of the theatre so that, when we need them, we are able to move around quickly and efficiently.
>
> [Scrub/Scout Nurse 3]

Discussion

In this study, huddles were an organizational response to a tragic event and in this example, an attempt to ensure that the exceptional, yet tragic event never happens again. From a resilience perspective, many organizational responses to critical incidents are fraught with problems (Hibbert et al. 2018; Hollnagel, Wears, and Braithwaite 2015); the introduction of new policies, Standardized Operating Procedures or checklists aims to limit variation but they are often additions to existing requirements, and in complex systems, they can make it more difficult for staff to do their work, or are simply not adhered to (Hollnagel, Wears, and Braithwaite 2015). However, the responses from OT management and staff examined here were relatively enlightened. Furthermore, huddles provided staff with greater scope to respond, monitor, learn and anticipate, and, therefore, in theory, fostered the OT's capacity for resilience.

The underlying mechanisms of huddles, in particular, have been argued to leverage key aspects of complex systems by focusing on meaningful conversations and relationships (Provost et al. 2015). In contested and busy healthcare settings, it is not enough to have these sorts of initiatives in place; they must be accepted and enacted by staff on the ground. Good communication and meaningful conversations are at the heart of a resilient approach.

Sustained in-depth data collection in the OT enabled us to identify the widespread use and clear value of the huddles among nursing staff. Moreover, being embedded in the OT for an extended period of time, first for observation work and then for interviews, provided the opportunity to both identify that these initiatives were taking place and develop trust with research participants for a full exploration of context and impact. Without trust, it seems unlikely that the interviewees would have provided so much detail on huddles, including how they enacted these initiatives and that they had been implemented in response to a critical incident. And yet, these insights were fundamental to more fully appreciate the system, its complexity and capacity for resilience.

This case offers a brief illustration of a process (huddles) that may contribute to OT resilience in the future. During the interviews, all participants mentioned that huddles were beneficial and provided them with structured, protected time to reflect and anticipate how their work would unfold, in addition to identifying potential problems and risks. However, due to patient privacy issues, we were unable to observe huddles as they took place, observation of which may have provided greater insight into the dynamics of the team (that is to say, how staff from different professional groups or levels of seniority interacted and the impact of this on ongoing behaviour and activity).

Finally, this case study derives from a larger international research project examining the management of OTs. As with the study of any applied setting that offers rich contextual detail, the intention is not only to publish further from these results but to feed results back to the OT staff. We believe that this will enable them to develop a greater understanding of their systems' capacity for resilience in line with four key resilience themes: to respond, monitor, learn and anticipate well.

Conclusion

In this study and presented in this chapter, we have examined how hospitals function as complex adaptive systems, and how staff expressed resilience in the face of a number of interlinked challenges. Resilience as a behaviour of such systems involves maintaining performance in the face of variable conditions. Although it can be difficult to directly observe resilience, in-depth qualitative methods, particularly sustained field observations and interviews, can assist in clarifying the characteristics of complex healthcare systems. Hollnagel's (2011) RAG framework – which involves responding, monitoring, learning and anticipating – provides a strategy for interpreting the capacity for resilience in complex systems. These issues were examined through a case study of an OT that experienced a critical incident and put in place safety huddles that arguably promote resilience and leverage complexity, rather than mandating more policies or thickening the rule book.

References

Allen, CR, DG Angeler, AS Garmestani, LH Gunderson, and CS Holling. 2014. "Panarchy: Theory and application." *Ecosystems* 17 (4):578–589. doi: 10.1007/s10021-013-9744-2.

Alonso, A, DP Baker, A Holtzman, R Day, H King, L Toomey, and E Salas. 2006. "Reducing medical error in the military health system: How can team training help?" *Human Resource Management Review* 16 (3):396–415.

Braithwaite, J, K Churruca, LA Ellis, J Long, R Clay-Williams, N Damen, . . . K Ludlow. 2017. *Complexity Science in Healthcare – Aspirations, Approaches, Applications and Accomplishments: A White Paper.* Sydney, Australia: Australian Institute of Health Innovation, Macquarie University.

Braithwaite, J, RL Wears, and E Hollnagel. 2015. "Resilient health care: Turning patient safety on its head." *International Journal for Quality in Health Care* 27 (5):418–420. doi: 10.1093/intqhc/mzv063.

Braithwaite, J, RL Wears, and E Hollnagel. 2016. *Resilient Health Care: Reconciling Work-as-Imagined and Work-as-Done.* Vol. 3. Boca Raton: CRC Press.

Braun, V, and V Clarke. 2006. "Using thematic analysis in psychology." *Qualitative Research in Psychology* 3 (2):77–101.

Cracknell, A, A Lovatt, A Winfield, S Arkhipkina, E McDonagh, A Green, and M Rooney. 2016. "Huddle up for safer healthcare: How frontline teams can work together to improve patient safety." *Future Hospital Journal* 3 (S2):S31–S31.

Demers, C. 2003. "L'entretien." In *Conduire un Projet de Recherche: Une perspective qualitative,* edited by Y Giordano. Paris: EMS.

Glymph, DC, M Olenick, S Barbera, EL Brown, L Prestianni, and C Miller. 2015. "Healthcare utilizing deliberate discussion linking events (HUDDLE): A systematic review." *AANA Journal* 83 (3):183–188.

Groleau, C. 2003. "L'observation." In *Conduire un Projet de Recherche: Une perspective qualitative,* edited by Y Giordano. Colombelles: Éditions EMS. 211–244.

Hibbert, PD, MJW Thomas, A Deakin, WB Runciman, J Braithwaite, S Lomax, . . . T Surwald. 2018. "Are root cause analyses recommendations effective and sustainable? An observational study." *International Journal for Quality in Health Care* 30 (2):124–131.

Hollnagel, E. 2010. "How resilient is your organisation? An introduction to the resilience analysis grid (RAG)." Sustainable Transformation: Building a resilient organization.

Hollnagel, E. 2011. "Epilogue: RAG – the resilience analysis grid." In *Resilience Engineering in Practice: A Guidebook,* edited by E Hollnagel, J Pariès, DD Woods, and J Wreathall. Farnham: Ashgate Publishing, Ltd. 275–296.

Hollnagel, E, J Braithwaite, and RL Wears. 2013. *Resilient Health Care.* Farnham: Ashgate Publishing, Ltd.

Hollnagel, E, J Braithwaite, and RL Wears. 2019. *Delivering Resilient Health Care.* London: Routledge.

Hollnagel, E, RL Wears, and J Braithwaite. 2015. "From safety-I to safety-II: A white paper." *The Resilient Health Care Net: University of Southern Denmark,* University of Florida, and Macquarie University, Australia.

Hollnagel, E, and DD Woods. 2006. "Epilogue: Resilience engineering precepts." In *Resilience Engineering: Concepts and Precepts.* Aldershot: Ashgate Publishing, Ltd. 347–358.

McDaniel Jr, RR, and DJ Driebe. 2001. "Complexity science and health care management." In *Advances in Health Care Management. Vol. 2, Advances in Health Care Management,* edited by LH Friedman, J Goes, and GT Savage. Bingley, UK: Emerald Group Publishing Limited. 11–36.

Morse, JM. 1995. *The Significance of Saturation*. Thousand Oaks: Sage.

New South Wales Auditor-General. 2013. *Managing Operating Theatre Efficiency for Elective Surgery*. Sydney, NSW: Audit Office of New South Wales.

NSW Agency for Clinical Innovation. 2014. "Operating theatre efficiency guidelines – a guide to the efficient management of operating theatres in New South Wales hospitals."

Provost, SM, HJ Lanham, LK Leykum, RR McDaniel Jr, and JA Pugh. 2015. "Health care huddles: Managing complexity to achieve high reliability." *Health Care Management Review* 40 (1):2–12. doi: 10.1097/HMR.0000000000000009.

Sheppard, F, M Williams, and VR Klein. 2013. "TeamSTEPPS and patient safety in healthcare." *Journal of Healthcare Risk Management* 32 (3):5–10.

Wacheux, F. 1996. *Méthodes Qualitatives et Recherche en Gestion*. Paris: Economica.

Wears, R, E Hollnagel, and J Braithwaite. 2015. *Resilient Health Care: The Resilience of Everyday Clinical Work*. Vol. 2. Farnham: Ashgate Publishing, Ltd.

Yin, RK. 2009. *Case Study Research: Design and Methods, Applied Social Research Methods Series*. Edited by RK Yin. 4th ed. Thousand Oaks: Sage.

Zhuravsky, L. 2019. "When Disaster Strikes: Sustained resilience performance in a clinical setting." In *Delivering Resilient Health Care*, edited by E Hollnagel, J Braithwaite, and RL Wears. Vol. IV. Abingdon: Taylor & Francis.

9 Qualitative assessment to improve everyday activities

Work-as-imagined and work-as-done

Robyn Clay-Williams, Elizabeth Austin, Jeffrey Braithwaite and Erik Hollnagel

Whether desiring to improve patient care, manage workplace processes, or determine what happened when something has gone awry, we must first understand what is happening in the workplace and how work is enacted on the frontlines of patient care when things go well. Patient care is delivered in a dynamic system, and clinicians must make continual small or large adjustments to accomplish everyday work. Those at a distance from the workplace, such as managers or system designers, are likely to take a broader view and thereby overlook the amount of necessary variation in the process of caring for patients. They are further displaced from the work (for example, in time, space or knowledge) and hence have a less accurate understanding about how it is done (Hollnagel 2015). As a result, work-as-done (WAD) when caring for patients can be very different to work-as-imagined (WAI) by those who manage or design healthcare systems (Braithwaite, Wears, and Hollnagel 2016). In this chapter, we will focus on the importance of understanding WAD, and illustrate it by comparing and contrasting WAI and WAD for a specific case.

So, how can we use qualitative methods to understand WAD, and how do we apply that understanding to design and implement new systems or system interventions? The 'gold standard' approach for understanding WAD is ethnographic observation (Nemeth and Herrera 2015), where one or more trained researchers are embedded in the workplace and observe how the work is enacted over time. Information on WAD can also be collected through interviews or focus groups with those who do the work, considering the subjective aspect of self-reporting. Traditional analyses of these qualitative ethnographic data through methods such as grounded theory or thematic analysis will yield important insights into WAD but will not necessarily identify the interdependencies between various tasks, the variation in how they are performed or the influence of time and the physical context on the processes that comprise everyday work. To enhance our level of understanding, we need to combine qualitative data collection and analysis methods with other data collection and analysis methods designed to capture the dynamic nature of activities, such as process mapping.

Process mapping is a useful method for understanding how work is enacted in the workplace and can be used for improving how work processes are implemented and investigating unwanted events, such as incidents or accidents. Tools that are traditionally used for process mapping, such as flowcharts, swim lane maps (Damelio 2011) or value stream maps (Rother and Shook 2003), can be very effective in mapping linear, technical systems but sometimes break down or fail to capture requisite richness when processes are more complex (for example, in areas such a healthcare, when process variability or adjustments form a normal and necessary part of everyday work). The Functional Resonance Analysis Method (FRAM) (Hollnagel 2012) has been specifically developed to describe processes in complex socio-technical systems. FRAM is a useful tool to help us understand WAD and to guide the design and implementation of new systems or processes. FRAM uses primarily qualitative data that is then used to construct a model of workplace processes and activities. FRAM produces a visual model to describe a task, in terms of the linked set of activities that make up that task.

The data for developing a FRAM model can be collected through any combination of ethnographic observations, interviews, focus groups and documented processes. Each activity (or 'function') is then described in terms of six aspects (see Figure 9.1):

1   Input (I) is what the function acts on or changes (an input is also used to start the function)

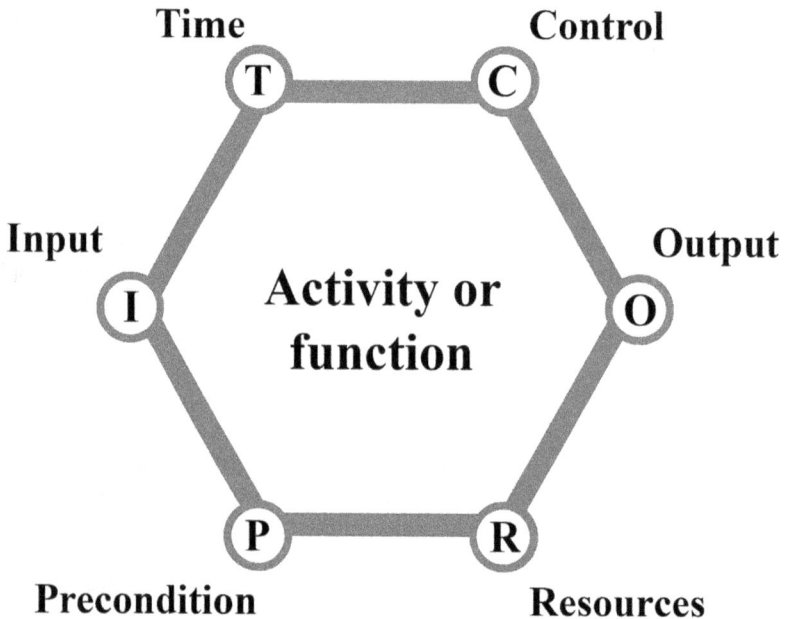

Figure 9.1 A FRAM activity (or function).

Source: Hollnagel, E. 2012. FRAM: *The Functional Resonance Analysis Method.* Farnham: Ashgate Publishing, Ltd.

2   Output (O) is what emerges from the function (this can be an outcome or a state change)
3   Precondition (P) is a condition that must be satisfied before the function can be commenced
4   Resources (R) are materials or people needed to carry out the function, or material consumed during the function
5   Control (C) is how the function is monitored or controlled
6   Time (T) refers to any time constraints that might affect completing the function

A FRAM model is created by mapping activities (functions) to show how the task is typically carried out, including where and how the activities depend on each other. It is a good idea to start at higher system levels where possible, and then drill down where needed, so that the resulting FRAM model is not overly crowded and remains a useful tool. A FRAM model of no more than 20 or so functions is a good indication that the chosen system level modelled is appropriate.

We can examine this by taking a look at a simple example from healthcare, the process of 'taking a blood sample' from a patient. The data for our example were collected as part of a project focusing on understanding current emergency department (ED) functioning in a large metropolitan public hospital in Australia. We sought to describe systemic constraints and identify tasks undertaken within the ED, including the different strategies individuals use to perform those tasks. Information was collected from publicly available documents relating to the work system (for example, policy documents and operating procedures), 263 hours of observations in the ED work setting and domain expert opinion (collected through walk/talk-throughs and/or interviews). These were reviewed to understand how functions are achieved in a public hospital ED. The process discussed here is the venepuncture process, as conducted by doctors in an ED setting.

Work-as-imagined

When characterizing WAI, we need to acknowledge the viewpoint of the manager, or person who has influence over the workplace design and resources. In the ED, venepuncture is governed through a number of regulatory processes. Guidelines for safe and high quality approaches to taking blood have been developed by the Australasian College for Emergency Medicine in conjunction with the Royal College of Pathologists of Australia (Australasian College for Emergency Medicine and the Royal College of Pathologists of Australia), the federal Department of Health (Pilbeam, Badrick, and Ridout 2013) and the Western Sydney Local Health District of which the hospital is a part (Hecimovic 2015). In addition, within the hospital, a Service Level Agreement has been developed between the ED and the hospital pathology laboratory (Australasian College for Emergency Medicine and the Royal College of Pathologists of Australia). Managers are likely to be aware of the existence of these guidelines but not the specific content.

There are three phases that comprise the collection and analysis of blood (Pilbeam, Badrick, and Ridout 2013). From initial collection up until the point that the blood is registered in the laboratory is called the pre-analytical phase; the analytical phase consists of the laboratory test process; and the post-analytical phase is where the doctor interprets the results and communicates them to the patient. Most errors have been found to occur during the pre-analytical phase (46–68.2% of total errors) (Dale and Novis 2002; Plebani 2006); our example explores this phase and offers thoughts as to why that might be so. The importance of training and competence alongside the example explored later has also been emphasized, particularly in relation to the pre-analytical phase (Pilbeam, Badrick, and Ridoutt 2013). However, in public hospitals, credentialed pathology collectors do not operate in the ED, mostly because of the unpredictable yet sometimes urgent need for blood collection and the 24-hour work cycle. Blood samples are therefore routinely collected by clinicians in the ED, primarily doctors. In Australia, a higher incidence of pre-analytical errors in samples collected from EDs has been found in samples collected by clinicians (doctors, nurses) or medical scientists (Pilbeam, Badrick, and Ridoutt 2013).

WAI is similar in concept to program theory, where it is assumed that the program's design and implementation will result in the desired outcomes (Funnell and Rogers 2011). Using program theory, a logic model of the process can be constructed. A logic model is a planning tool to simplify and illustrate the process e.g. a flow chart. Managers would not normally consult hospital documents that discuss the blood collection process in great detail. Using information from the governance documents applicable to our study ED (Australasian College for Emergency Medicine and the Royal College of Pathologists of Australia, Pilbeam, Badrick, and Ridoutt 2013) and discussion with hospital managers, a typical logic model of the pre-analytical phase of the venepuncture process, which consists of writing a referral, taking blood and dispatching the sample to the pathology laboratory, was created (as shown in Figure 9.2).

We can also construct a FRAM model of the WAI version of the venepuncture process. This is shown in Figure 9.3 and consists of the same three primary functions as the logic model: 1) write the referral, 2) take the blood and 3) send the blood to the pathology laboratory. The FRAM model, however, provides additional information to the logic model: we can see that the referral function, for example, rather than being an input to taking the blood, is actually a precondition to sending the blood to the pathology laboratory, meaning that the referral does not have to be completed before the venepuncture commences.

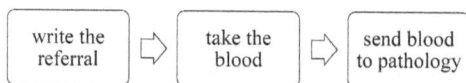

Figure 9.2 Pre-analytical phase: Taking a blood sample – logic model.
Source: Authors' own work.

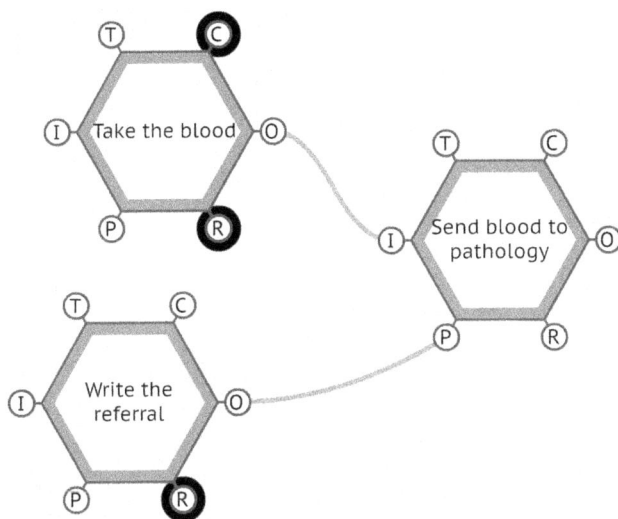

Figure 9.3 Pre-analytical phase: Taking a blood sample work-as-imagined.

Source: Authors' own work.

In a FRAM model, a highlighted circle around an aspect of a function indicates that this aspect has not yet been fully accounted for. For example, we can see in Figure 9.3 that there is a Resource for 'write the referral', for example, which in this case is the availability of a computer. There are Controls for the 'take the blood' action, which in this case are the applicable guidelines or protocols for taking blood and the need for the doctor to be trained in the correct process. There is also a Resource associated with 'take the blood' – in this case, the blood kit that contains the cannula, tourniquet and blood sample containers. From the view of the manager, taking a blood sample looks like a very simple process involving only three steps. In WAI, the only critical issues to consider are that the doctor has access to a computer to write the referral, one or more protocols must be written and maintained, and that sufficient blood kits are supplied to meet patient demand. When laying out the ED for the WAI version of this process, a system designer would position the blood dispatch tube close to the location where the blood is taken, and perhaps feel that they have optimized the process.

Work-as-done

Based on 110 hours observing doctors in the ED, we constructed a FRAM model of WAD in 'taking a blood sample'. The FRAM model is actually comprised of a minimum of 12 discrete tasks, as shown in Figure 9.4: 1) obtain the blood sampling kit, 2) put on gloves, 3) wipe the patient's skin with a sterile pad, 4) apply the

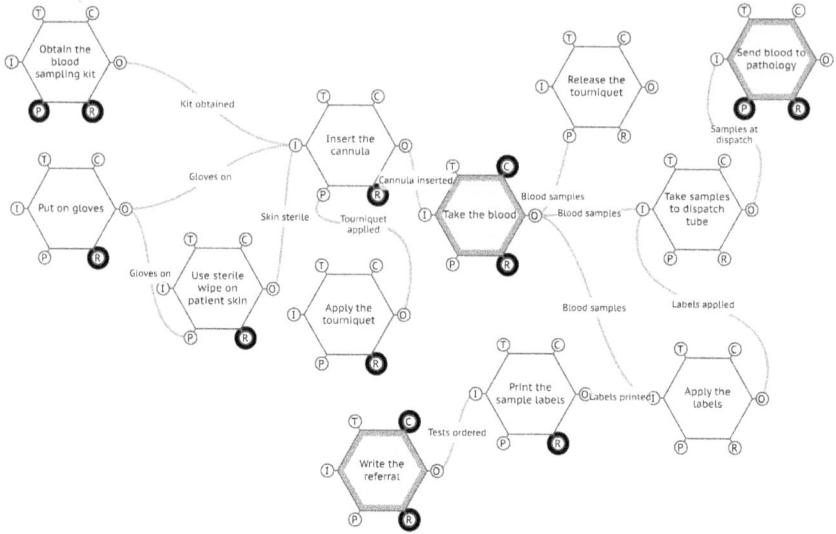

Figure 9.4 Pre-analytical phase: Taking a blood sample work-as-done.

Source: Authors' own work.

tourniquet, 5) insert the cannula, 6) take the blood, 7) release the tourniquet, 8) write the referral, 9) print the test labels, 10) apply the labels, 11) take the test samples to the pneumatic dispatch tube and 12) send the blood samples to pathology. The three steps in the WAI model are still there (highlighted), but we now get a sense of the complexity of the process from the WAD viewpoint. Not only are there many more steps or functions, but some of the steps are in a different order to what we anticipated from the WAI model, some steps are dependent on each other (see steps with Preconditions) and there are many more specific Resources required than just the blood sampling kit.

To take this simple example further, what can we now learn from the WAD FRAM model that would not have been evident from the WAI version? Let's start with the first part of the process, up to the point where the cannula is inserted (expanded in Figure 9.5). Beginning with the step 'obtain the blood sampling kit', we have the same blood kit Resource indicated as in the WAI model, but there is also a Precondition that the relevant trolley (of which there are many in an ED) be pre-stocked with an appropriate kit. We can also see from Figure 9.5 that there are a number of paths to inserting the cannula. The ideal path, based on documented guidelines, would be to: 1) obtain the blood sampling kit, 2) put on gloves, 3) use a sterile wipe to clean the patient's skin (putting on gloves is a Precondition, to ensure that the patient's skin is not contaminated) and 4) insert the cannula. There are three inputs to the 'insert the cannula' function, however, which means that in addition to the ideal path there are two alternate paths: the kit could be obtained and the cannula inserted without the patient's skin being

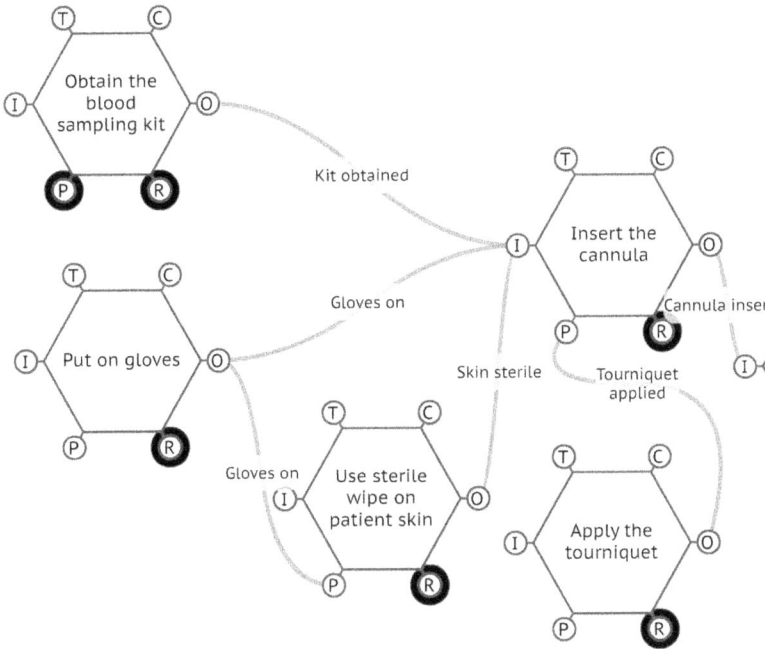

Figure 9.5 Pre-analytical phase: Taking a blood sample work-as-done – inserting the cannula.

Source: Authors' own work.

cleaned using a sterile wipe, or without the doctor wearing gloves. The 'use sterile wipe on patient skin' is what is known as a 'hidden function' (Hollnagel 2012), as it can be bypassed by moving directly from 'put on gloves' to 'insert the cannula'. Hidden functions indicate something that can go awry, particularly when the doctor is rushed, as hidden functions are not Preconditions for future functions and bypassing them saves time (Hollnagel 2012).

Moving further into the process (expanded in Figure 9.6), we can see that 'take the blood' is a Precondition to 'release the tourniquet'. But as there are no following functions to this task, it would be possible to forget to release the tourniquet and the error not to be picked up. While this may seem unlikely, we know that doctors in EDs are interrupted in 11% of all tasks and, when interrupted, fail to return to 18.5% of those tasks (Westbrook et al. 2010). We observed, for example, that sometimes a patient had to remind the doctor to remove the tourniquet after the blood had been taken and the doctor was about to leave the room.

The path that begins with writing the referral, which then generates labels to be printed and affixed to the samples, has a number of additional steps to the referral writing function from the WAI viewpoint. We found this to be a significant source of delay to the overall process: there were sometimes insufficient computers

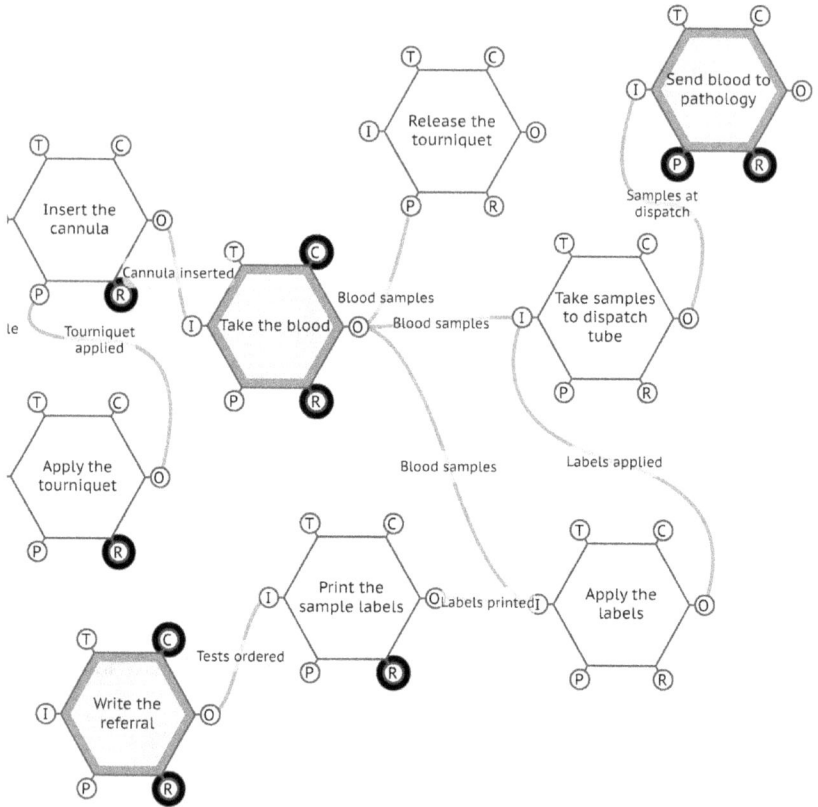

Figure 9.6 Pre-analytical phase: Taking a blood sample work-as-done – preparing samples for dispatch.

Source: Authors' own work.

for the number of doctors, particularly around handover time when there was a 2-hour overlap between shifts, the computers that were available sometimes froze or would not link to the label printer, and the printer sometimes refused to function or ran out of labels. If the label printer malfunctioned, the doctor would make a phone call to the pathology lab to ask them to send a re-print request to the printer in the ED. This in itself is a 'workaround': if the doctor sought to initiate a re-print from the ED, they would have to cancel and reorder the requested blood tests on the computer. Sometimes the printed labels did not include all the requested tests, and these had to be hand-written onto the printed labels.

'Apply the labels' is another hidden function – the blood samples could be taken directly to the dispatch tube and dispatched without the labels attached. For experienced ED doctors, the 'take blood' scenario is so common that many of these steps have become habitual, but for junior doctors who are less familiar with the process, sending the samples off without labelling is distinctly possible.

The FRAM model is also able to show where processes are variable in the time they take to perform. This variability can result from technological, human or organizational factors. Functions that are delayed or take longer than expected cause delays in the downstream functions. Where multiple paths occur in parallel, delays in one path can result in downstream functions performed out of order, particularly if a downstream activity can be initiated by more than one input. The functions that are determined to be variable are indicated by a sine curve inside the hexagon (Figure 9.7).

Variability was identified in three functions. First, the time to obtain the blood sampling kit can be variable: the blood kits are not pre-assembled, as the components are dependent on the characteristics of the patient (e.g., size of the cannula) and their presenting illness (e.g., type of sample container, number of sample containers). In WAD, the closest trolley might contain some parts of the kit but other elements, particularly if the patient is not typical (e.g., small child, someone with difficult-to-access veins), may need to be sourced from other trolleys located elsewhere in the ED or the storeroom.

Second, the 'insert the cannula' function is variable in the time it takes to insert the cannula depending on the patient characteristics (e.g., intravenous drug user with damaged veins, older person with low blood pressure, patient with needle phobia) and the experience of the doctor. Third, the 'send blood to pathology'

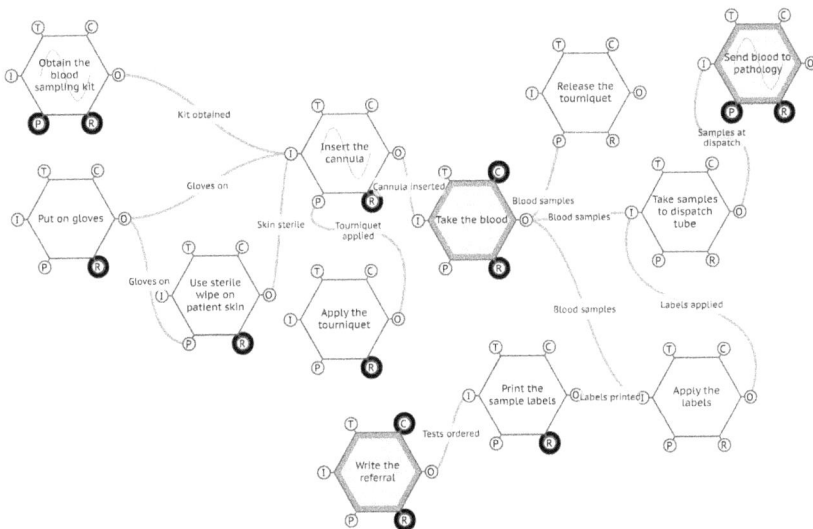

Figure 9.7 Pre-analytical phase: Taking a blood sample work-as-done – showing variable functions.

Source: Authors' own work.

function, which is a matter of bagging the samples, putting them into a pneumatic canister and sending the canister down a tube, appears to be straightforward but was also highly variable in terms of time. There was a Precondition that the pneumatic tube be functional (it failed multiple times over the two weeks of our observations) and a Resource in the form of the canister to transport the samples (sometimes three canisters were available, ready to use, in the basket, but just as often there were none, and the samples could not be immediately sent and were left on top of the tube dispatch box while the doctors went about other business).

Looking at the 'taking blood' process overall we have the numerous Resources that are essential to perform the task, most of which were not identified in the WAI model: blood kit (with variable components), gloves of varying sizes and type, sterile wipes, cannulas of varying sizes, tourniquets, access to the computer, a functioning printer, blank sample labels, canisters to send the samples down the tube to pathology and a functioning pneumatic tube. Over the 110-hour observation period, each of these resources was observed to be missing or unavailable when needed on one or more occasions.

The additional detail and insight provided by the WAD FRAM model is helpful in understanding how clinicians do their work, and the constraints that they face, even in a simple task such as 'taking blood'. The use of the FRAM to identify differences between WAI and WAD can have consequences for design, work management and investigations. Outlining the differences between WAI and WAD through FRAM modelling can inform system design. For example, the 'taking blood' FRAM model could be used to inform changes to the IT system, cannula kit and the placement of resources. FRAM models can also provide insight into work management, identifying functions that could be aligned with the evolving demands of clinical practice, and those that could be updated to improve work management. Finally, mapping the difference between WAI and WAD using the FRAM can guide investigations of when things go wrong, highlighting steps in a task where variation, preconditions and hidden functions occur in WAD.

Discussion and conclusion

We have shown through a simple example how FRAM can be used to understand WAD as well as identify areas where WAI differs from WAD. We can see that modelling WAD provides us with considerably more information than is available from a WAI perspective. Establishing the presence of hidden functions and multiple starting triggers for activities can also help explain why things that normally go right can sometimes go wrong. Armed with this understanding, managers or system designers can then describe and implement system improvements that are better matched to the physical and cognitive needs of the humans who are doing the work. When laying out an ED for the WAD process, for example, the system designer must consider the locations of the trolleys, computers, printers and so on rather than just the locations for taking and dispatching the blood.

The FRAM can be used at different granularities (macro-, meso- or micro-), depending on the question of interest. Internationally, FRAM has been used as a tool to understand the gap between WAI and WAD in healthcare (Damen et al. 2018; Raben et al. 2018). For example, FRAM has been used to map the division of tasks among clinical disciplines in the management of preoperative anticoagulation (Damen et al. 2018), and to process map the early detection of sepsis (Raben et al. 2018). FRAM has also been used to design new healthcare processes where WAI and WAD are better aligned (Clay-Williams, Hounsgaard, and Hollnagel 2015; Ross et al. 2018). For example, to model workflow in a clinical setting to develop and implement guidelines (Clay-Williams, Hounsgaard, and Hollnagel 2015), and to develop recommendations for system-wide interventions in the context of fluoride application (Ross et al. 2018). FRAM is a flexible tool that allows researchers, managers and system designers to examine work processes at different levels of a system and identify areas where WAI and WAD can be better aligned.

Designing systems that take into account how work is done reduces the need for user 'workarounds' and therefore makes work less variable. Qualitative data collection allows us to capture how work is performed on the frontlines of patient care as well as how work is imagined in guidelines and protocols. FRAM produces a visual model describing work processes in terms of the linked set of activities that make up the process and can be developed for processes at all levels of a system. Developing FRAM models based on qualitative data helps us to understand WAD, identify the differences between WAI and WAD, and to guide the design and implementation of new processes at multiple levels of systems.

References

Australasian College for Emergency Medicine and the Royal College of Pathologists of Australia. Guideline: Pathology Testing in the Emergency Department in *February 2013 (RCPA) March 2013 (ACEM), Revised July 2018 (RCPA) December 2018 (ACEM); 1/2013 (RCPA) G125 (ACEM).*

Braithwaite, J, RL Wears, and E Hollnagel. 2016. *Resilient Health Care: Reconciling Work-as-Imagined and Work-as-Done.* Vol. 3. Boca Raton: CRC Press.

Clay-Williams, R, J Hounsgaard, and E Hollnagel. 2015. "Where the rubber meets the road: Using FRAM to align work-as-imagined with work-as-done when implementing clinical guidelines." *Implementation Science* 10 (1):125.

Dale, JC, and DA Novis. 2002. "Outpatient phlebotomy success and reasons for specimen rejection: A Q-probes study." *Archives of Pathology & Laboratory Medicine* 126 (4):416–419.

Damelio, R. 2011. *The Basics of Process Mapping.* New York: Productivity Press.

Damen, NL, M Moesker, J Braithwaite, J Kaplan, J Hamming, and R Clay-Williams. 2018. "Preoperative anticoagulation management in everyday clinical practice: An international comparative analysis of work-as-done using the functional resonance analysis method." *Journal of Patient Safety,* July 7, 2018, publish ahead of print. doi: 10.1097/ PTS.0000000000000515.

Funnell, SC, and PJ Rogers. 2011. *Purposeful Program Theory: Effective Use of Theories of Change and Logic Models.* Vol. 31. San Francisco: John Wiley & Sons, Ltd.

Hecimovic, M. 2015. *Venepuncture Handbook.* Sydney, Australia: Institute of Clinical Pathology and Medical Research, Pathology West – Westmead.

Hollnagel, E. 2012. FRAM: *The Functional Resonance Analysis Method*. Farnham: Ashgate Publishing, Ltd.

Hollnagel, E. 2015. "Why is work-as-imagined different to work-as-done?" In *Resilient Health Care: The Resilience of Everyday Clinical Work*, edited by R Wears, E Hollnagel, and J Braithwaite. Vol. 2. Farnham: Ashgate Publishing, Ltd. 249–264.

Nemeth, CP, and I Herrera. 2015. "Building change: Resilience engineering after ten years." *Reliability Engineering & System Safety* 141 (September):1–4.

Pilbeam, V, T Badrick, and L Ridoutt. 2013. *Best Practice Pathology Collection*. Canberra, Australia: Department of Health.

Plebani, M. 2006. "Errors in clinical laboratories or errors in laboratory medicine?" *Clinical Chemistry and Laboratory Medicine (CCLM)* 44 (6):750–759.

Raben, DC, B Viskum, KL Mikkelsen, J Hounsgaard, SB Bogh, and E Hollnagel. 2018. "Application of a non-linear model to understand healthcare processes: Using the functional resonance analysis method on a case study of the early detection of sepsis." *Reliability Engineering & System Safety* 177:1–11.

Ross, A, A Sherriff, J Kidd, W Gnich, J Anderson, L Deas, and L Macpherson. 2018. "A systems approach using the functional resonance analysis method to support fluoride varnish application for children attending general dental practice." *Applied Ergonomics* 68:294–303.

Rother, M, and J Shook. 2003. *Learning to See: Value Stream Mapping to add Value and Eliminate Muda*. Cambridge, MA: Lean Enterprise Institute.

Westbrook, JI, A Woods, MI Rob, WT Dunsmuir, and RO Day. 2010. "Association of interruptions with an increased risk and severity of medication administration errors." *Archives of Internal Medicine* 170 (8):683–690.

10 Narrativizing cancer patients' longitudinal experiences of care

Qualitative inquiry into lived and online melanoma stories

Klay Lamprell, Frances Rapport and Jeffrey Braithwaite

Introduction

Qualitative research methodologies offer portals into patients' experiences of care. They seek out the myriad ways that interactions and processes in healthcare systems can enhance, or diminish, a patient's quality of life. They offer opportunities to investigate and conceptualize the personal nature of patient experience. In this chapter we discuss a qualitative methodology for investigating and theorizing the experiences of patients as they move from diagnosis to outcome – the patient journey (Lamprell and Braithwaite 2016).

Our research centred on the longitudinal healthcare experiences of people with melanoma, which is a malignant, aggressive, heterogeneous form of skin cancer that is increasing in incidence and prevalence throughout the world (Thompson, Scolyer, and Kefford 2005; Apalla et al. 2017). We wanted to characterize the pivotal points of tension and transition through clinical phases and across healthcare settings from patients' perspectives, since they are the only people who see (and experience in their bodies and their minds) the whole journey (Ben-Tovim et al. 2008).

We faced two sets of decisions when designing the project, which we summarize here and then explore in more detail. The first decision was related to the value of the longitudinal research we wanted to do. Qualitative longitudinal research (QLR) (Holland, Thomson, and Henderson 2006) using a trajectory approach is uncommon in healthcare research settings (Grossoehme and Lipstein 2016), largely because it is time-consuming and logistically challenging, given that healthcare systems in real world terms are a complex, fractured and often vaguely conjoined set of healthcare services (Braithwaite 2018). Additionally, QLR produces a large quantity of rich data to analyze (Calman, Brunton, and Molassiotis 2013). We needed to consider its merit over other forms of investigation for our research in this context, such as the periodic, short-answer questionnaire survey (Tsianakas et al. 2012).

The second problem we faced was methodological. Through the collection of narrative data and thematic modes of data analysis we could identify melanoma patients' perceptions of care at temporal points in their clinical trajectory

(Braun, Clarke, and Rance 2014). We wanted, as well, to capture and represent the dynamic, transitory nature of patient experience across a medical journey as patients live it and tell it (Mattingly 1998). In context to their unfolding life and death drama (Frank 2013; Hurwitz and Charon 2013), the disruption – and for some, chaos – of cancer coexists with an overarching view of the clinical journey as a purposeful, hopeful movement towards survival. Progressive healthcare events and interactions with healthcare professionals hold greater and lesser significance as points of tension and transition within that overall narrative. While temporality is privileged in QLR (Thomson and McLeod 2015), there is no methodology by which to characterize the interconnectedness and relativity of patients' perceptions of healthcare experiences across their medical journeys.

The value proposition

Melanoma is most often attributed to the exposure of skin to ultraviolet radiation, in particular from the sun, (Panther and Brodland 2019) though some 5 percent of cases develop melanoma in other tissues, such as the eyes (Chattopadhyay et al. 2016). Early detection and surgical excision with adequate margins significantly improve chances of survivorship (Walter et al. 2014). However, people who have been treated for one melanoma are between nine and up to 16 (McLoone et al. 2013; Miller et al. 2016) times more likely than the general population to develop another primary melanoma, amplifying the need for periodic clinical surveillance for recurrence or metastases (Trotter et al. 2013). Advanced stages of the disease (e.g., Stage 4, when it has spread to other organs) are considered incurable (Hill et al. 2015) and therapeutic options may be limited or even futile (Thompson, Scolyer, and Kefford 2005). Disfigurement and disability from surgery may institute a set of additional medical and psychological threats and deeply-rooted traumas as well as other physical, social and emotional impacts that require ongoing management (Palesh et al. 2014). Every instance of the disease establishes an acute – and then ever-present – need for services from healthcare organizations (Cornish et al. 2009).

Knowledge of the whole journey, from the patient's perspective, can help healthcare systems prepare for that chronic load. Characterizing the longitudinal experience of clinical care for these patients allows insights into the events, or sets of events, that are pivotal points of need for supportive care during that journey. This knowledge of where to fortify resources in the multi-service narrative of patient experience is key to building proactive pathways of care. Proactivity is the hallmark of system resilience in the face of "irreconcilable goals – customer demands, performance pressures, work and workforce stresses, and cost challenges" (Wears, Hollnagel, and Braithwaite 2015, xxi). Building resilience requires that we should "pay attention to how clinical care can be supported so that the number of intended and acceptable outcomes becomes as high as possible" (Braithwaite, Wears, and Hollnagel 2015, 419).

This is the value rationale we took into the project: that longitudinal, qualitative knowledge of melanoma patients' experiences of care can inform the enactment of resilience within healthcare organizations and across systems of care. Our objective was to understand which experiences of care are of greater and lesser consequence to patients as they move through their hopeful journeys towards survival. To give substance and form to this perspective requires more than cross-sectional 'snapshot views'.

Methodological design

Many qualitative methodologies rely on descriptive accounts – a rendering of subjective evidence of experience. They take as their basic premise that the experience of another can only be known through the narration (or other presentational form, such as a visual presentation which may be supported by narration) of their experience, and so the capacity to describe aspects and properties of experience can translate "knowing into telling" (White 1980, 5). We set out to collect narrative data on patients' journeys by interviewing and shadowing a group of people with melanoma, and by analyzing extant online stories written by people with melanoma.

As noted, however, we struggled to identify an approach to data analysis that would serve our research question (Connelly and Clandinin 1990). Here we were at a crossroads that was first articulated by cognitive psychologist Jerome Bruner (1986) and subsequently re-articulated by Donald Polkinghorne (1995) amongst others. "Paradigmatic-type narrative inquiry" (Polkinghorne 1995, 5) deconstructs narrative accounts of experience in order to identify, classify and generalize significant elements. It is the mode of inquiry most often employed in social science by anthropologists and sociologists for example and creates thematic *categories*. Narrative-type narrative inquiry investigates elements of experience, such as events, thoughts and feelings, as they occur in a framework of emplotted *story*. Emplotment configures experience as a dynamic progression from a starting situation or problem towards resolution or "clarification" (Polkinghorne 1995, 7). It is the mode of inquiry employed commonly by psychologists and historians and a means of representing experience widely used by writers.

Our endeavor aimed to bring together thematic *categories* and emplotted *story*. Our resolution was to build on the established idea of a 'grand' narrative or archetypal plot of illness journey (Frank 2012, 2013; Smith and Sparkes 2008). We approached the grand plot as a heuristic for understanding the implications of progressive events of melanoma patient experience generalized across multiple patient perspectives. Using this heuristic, categories of subjectively consequential events and situations could be interpreted as pivotal transitions for patients in their overall stories.

The seminal work of Arthur Frank in the narrative theory of illness identified three core ways in which the survival plot is played out by people with life-threatening sickness: as a hopeful movement towards approximate restitution of life before illness; as a transformational progression towards a new outlook and purpose gained from the suffering; or as a desired escape from the chaos that the disruption of illness has wrought (Frank 2013, 2012). These archetypal plots

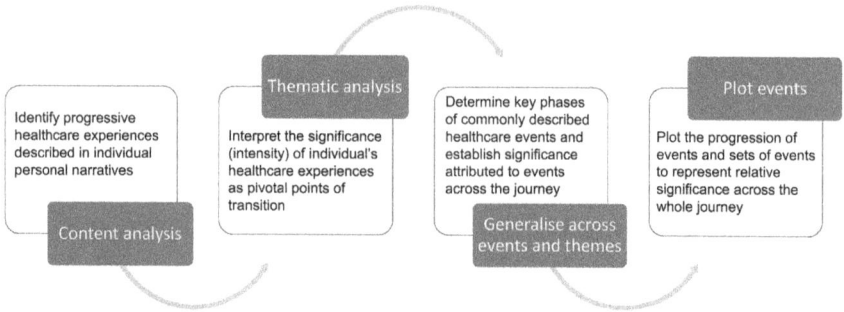

Figure 10.1 Method of analysis for narrativizing patient journey.
Source: Authors' own work.

theorize the ways that personal identity fundamentally frames perceptions of illness journeys. Our aim was to conceptualize the ways that progressive events of care foundationally shape overall experiences of clinical trajectories. The process we decided on is represented in Figure 10.1.

Pathways to addressing the problem

We applied this approach to two extant studies of melanoma patients. In one study, which we call Project A, seven people with advanced and metastatic melanoma attending a medical oncology clinic at a large, public tertiary referral centre in Sydney, Australia, were progressively shadowed and interviewed by one researcher over a ten-month period (Lamprell, Chin, and Braithwaite 2019). In the other study, which we call Project B, we considered 214 personal stories from authors of online autobiographical accounts of melanoma, published in the personal story sections of melanoma and cancer support websites. We characterized the two studies as *lived* and *online* ethnography (Lamprell and Braithwaite 2018).

Project A: lived ethnography

The participant population for this study was small to enable in-depth interviewing and close shadowing. Of the nine people who agreed to take part, two died before the study began. Table 10.1 describes the patient population participant to the study.

The settings for interviews with the participants and observations of their interactions with the supervising oncologist and other oncology specialists included: clinical consultation rooms, hospital administration and reception areas, a diagnostic imaging clinic, an oncology treatment centre, a radiology department, a general hospital ward, car parks and cafes within the hospital precinct and one participant's home (in response to his preference for this environment).

Table 10.1 Participants' demographic profiles and health histories

Partici-pant	Gender	Age*	Stage¹	Melanoma/tumour	Length of time since previous melanoma	How latest diagnosis occurred
PA	F	75+	4	Lungs, stomach, skull and brain	20 years	After weeks of becoming forgetful and confused, PA suffered stroke-like symptoms and was taken to hospital where investigations led to the identification of tumours
PB	M	75+	4	Left leg lymph nodes, lung	12 years	Ultrasound for deep vein thrombosis (DVTs) identified enlarged lymph glands
PC	M	25+	3–4	Right arm Lymph nodes	2 months	Enlarged lymph nodes were identified in first surveillance scan after melanoma on back had been excised
PD	F	65+	4	Stomach, lung, liver	4.5 years	Fell at home, taken to hospital, investigations led to the identification of tumours
PE	M	85+	1/4	Eye	N/A	Scheduled cataract examination identified lump
PF	M	70+	4	Rib, spine, kidney	2 years	Investigation of ongoing pain from broken rib led to the identification of tumours
PG	M	70+	4	Lung, pancreas	4 years	Investigation of abdominal pain led to the identification of tumours

1 Tumor, Node, Metastasis (TNM) staging system classifies cancer stages according to an alphanumeric system.
 Table Caption: '+' = a five-year variance

Source: Lamprell, K, M Chin, and J Braithwaite. 2019. "'Can I still get a tattoo?" Patients' experiences across the clinical trajectory for metastatic melanoma: a dynamic narrative model of patient journey." *Patient Experience Journal* 6 (1):87–93.

All interviews were conducted in person initially, and then, progressively, they involved phone, Skype and email correspondence as multiple data capture events that embellished understanding.

The data collection process mapped to the chronological framework of the patients' pathways and included diagnostic, administrative, therapeutic and social welfare events. Purposeful interviews ensured wide-ranging perceptions could be captured across specialty groups and clinical expertise, while also drawing patient participants into descriptions of events that occurred outside the 'ethnographic zone'. These events included lead-up to diagnosis that occurred before the research began and patients' experiences of treatment for comorbidities alongside the main melanoma treatment pathway.

Initial help-seeking for most of the patient participants was not defined in terms of skin problems. Advanced and metastatic melanoma can present differently to primary melanomas and the first symptoms of illness, for the majority of patient participants, occurred in a context of severe pain or significant dysfunction. The urgency of identifying the problem shaped patients' perceptions of the events of care.

Once diagnosed, patients were able to conceive an overarching plot to their journeys. The prognosis for people with advanced or metastatic melanoma is poor and taking action did not always mean receiving treatment. Indeed, for some participants pain relief took precedence and for one, death was welcome. For those who could receive treatment, experiences of care were given more or less consequence in relation to needs for information provision and preferences in decision-making as well as support for adaptation to the collateral 'damage' of radiation, surgery and chemotherapy.

The few participants who eventually entered a 'new normal' of therapeutic regimes and surveillance programs viewed their patient journeys as ongoing and circular: every ailment was a potential indicator of a metastases necessitating urgent medical attention. Overall, it was their "enfolding of a generative past and a future potential in the present moment, and not the location of that moment in any abstract chronology" (Ingold 2011, 74) that defined their experience of their journey.

Project B: online ethnography

We had limited control over 'recruitment' of the second patient population, the online group. A sampling frame could not be determined because the data were unsolicited and demographic information was generally not supplied. Specifics on gender, age, location and type of staging of their melanomas were embedded in some of these patient accounts but not all. We accepted these limitations and focused our selection criteria on levels of ethical governance by host websites and the narrative authenticity of the accounts published on those sites, excluding, for example, accounts written as evaluations of specific healthcare organizations. Table 10.2 describes the final scope of the study.

Table 10.2 Scope of study

Population size	283 stories identified as meeting the inclusion criteria; 214 selected for data collection.
Territory	Not limited to politically bounded territories but collected from English language websites.
Demographics	Author's gender was the only consistently available demographic characteristic. Of the 214 stories there were 149 female authors, 64 male authors and one whose gender could not be determined.
Date	Publication dates and dates of illness experiences were not consistently available. From available information, the publication dates ranged from 2008 to 2016.
Health status	Information on the clinical staging of melanoma was inconsistent within and between stories.

Ethnographic immersion in these lives comprised iterative layers of affiliation, beginning with simple readings and note-taking and leading to deep analysis within, and meta-analysis across, their accounts. Three defining periods of medical management emerged: 1) lead-up to diagnosis; 2) diagnosis, treatment and recovery; and 3) post treatment and recurrence. Detailed descriptions of events within these periods provided an imaginative journey into a storied world of interactions with doctors and other healthcare professionals, tests, surgeries, radiation, chemotherapy, palliative care and follow-up care.

The richness of these narrations exposed multiple layers of cognition about, and responsiveness to, healthcare experiences. Events were contextualized in terms of the quality of medicine being practiced and received, participants' satisfaction with services, the implications of particular events for the ultimate goal of survival and also the repercussions of healthcare events for friends and family, careers, day-to-day functionality, finances, and own and others' existential philosophies on life.

The people, places and values that mattered to the contributors often featured as 'through-lines' in the accounts, introduced early in the narrative – or in a prologue to the narrative – as part of an exposition of life before melanoma and then drawn through the telling of the journey. The journey was nearly always positioned as a life narrative starting in an ordinary life-world, shifting into the often protracted period during which symptoms were recognized, moving onto the sometimes convoluted pathways that led to diagnosis, traveling through the acute clinical trajectory of care and arriving at an arbitrary point of completion. The end of the account was not always the resolution of overarching goals since the medical journey was often far from over, but commonly the accounts used the narrative device of epilogue to convey some kind of conclusion (Lamprell and Braithwaite 2019).

It became apparent that while the diagnosis of melanoma was of itself a point of great tension, the investigative events taking place just after diagnosis – to determine staging of the melanoma for example – were the highest points of tension and transition across the patient journey, both for first and subsequent diagnoses. The events of this period caused the greatest vulnerability because results would determine next courses of action, forms of surgery and/or chemical treatments and, ultimately, the likelihood of survival. The decisions made at this time would inform so many aspects of these people's lives, from relationships to work to everyday logistics and functionality.

Discussion

In this section we offer an aggregate view of the findings of Projects A and B (see Tables 10.3, 10.4, 10.5 and 10.6), describing the key sets of events, perspectives and experiences that were identified in each of the two data sources. We then model a generalized plot of the patient journey for each patient population.

While each patient's narrative of events comprised "singular, irreplicable or incommensurable" (Charon 2008, 45) goals, the heuristic of modelling a generalized plot for each set of findings resulted in two very different schemas of how melanoma patients collectively experienced their journeys. The meta-narrative model for participants in the lived ethnography (Figure 10.2) features a circular plot, representing the experience of survivors that their clinical trajectory for melanoma is never-ending. The pivotal transitions of this plot are located between phases of patient experience comprising grouped sets of events.

Table 10.3 First phase of the patient journey: A comparison of thematic findings from two data sources

	PROJECT A: *Ethnographic study of people with melanoma*	PROJECT B: *Written personal accounts of melanoma*
Patient-led delays	Project A: 'Initiation' Rationalization of health disturbances e.g., thinking a health issue is 'just stress' or too much going on in life, waiting for an upcoming appointment. Having been told pain is normal for a particular health condition. Low sensitivity to or awareness of melanoma recurrence and perception of being 'clear' of melanoma.	Project B: 'Lead-up to diagnosis' Rationalization of health disturbances and pain e.g., serious illness is 'something that happens to someone else' or 'too busy'. Incompatibility of own skin changes in comparison with pictures shown in melanoma awareness campaigns.
Clinician-led delays	Low healthcare provider awareness of risk of recurrence.	Wait times for specialist appointment. Missed diagnoses. Conflict between patient and physician about the need for further investigation of a symptom.

Table 10.4 Second phase of the patient journey: A comparison of thematic findings from two data sources

Project A: 'Identification'		*Project B: 'Diagnosis, treatment and recovery'*	
Impact of investigations and consultations	Significant logistical and time commitment in appointments. Infection and pain from open lung biopsy. Physical difficulties getting to appointments and managing movement during scans. Appreciation of scans and consultations scheduled to occur in the one location or on the one day.	Co-ordination of healthcare services	Appreciation of coordination of appointments made for tests, consultations with oncologists and surgeons, and surgery.
Information pathways and knowledge absorption about diagnosis	Appreciation of detailed explanations of scanning equipment and visually represented results. Confusion about names and functions of types of scans. Difficulties of staying focused during consultations. Reliance on information provided by hospital and clinicians. Concern with the negative implications of 'knowing too much'.		
Impacts of diagnosis	Desire to be given a timeframe for survival. Frustration at clinicians' explanations of prognosis as complex. Impact related to expectations of recurrence e.g., some expecting a recurrence, others shocked. Surprise at the role of 'luck' in finding the melanomas. Confusion when tumours were assumed to be melanoma but could not be confirmed.	Impact of news of the diagnosis	Impact of communication with clinic receptionists to organize test result appointments. Physician choices in tone and wording in delivery of test results. Negative impact of contrast between earlier reassurance and subsequent diagnosis. Emotional and physiological impact of news depending on physician style and tone. Impact of hearing a diagnosis on the capacity to absorb information about diagnosis and treatment options.

Table 10.5 Third phase of the patient journey: A comparison of thematic findings from two data sources

Project A: 'Action'		Project B: 'Diagnosis, treatment and recovery'	
Information pathways	Vague understanding of the BRAF[1] concept and what testing or results means. Appreciation for pamphlets about treatment. Appreciation of tours of chemo-therapy clinics.	Information pathways	Need for more information about the likely effects of chemical therapies. Concern with lack of preparation for clinical trials.
Treatment decisions	Preference for non-collaborative decision-making; physicians asked to make the choice. Decision to 'do what it takes'. Going into clinical trials for the sake of future generations and need to be proactive in sourcing clinical trials. Want physicians to make decisions. Make strategic choices in healthcare providers then do what they say. Decision limbo until BRAF test results come back causes frustration. Consideration of second opinion on treatment options.	Treatment decision	Desire for help in finding, understanding and making decisions about alternative treatment options.
Physical and psychosocial experiences of treatment	Rationalization of side effects in light of the 'end-goal'. Concern about mentioning side effects in case taken off treatment or removed from clinical trial. Significant side effects in clinical trial and need to embark on second trial for drug to manage side effects. Scheduled chemo-treatments become routine and relationships are developed with clinic staff. Significant logistical and time commitment in attending clinical trial over years.	Surgery and recovery	Frustration at long wait times for surgery. Shock about the size and impact of the surgical excisions. Surprise at the complexity of the recovery process. Frustration and concern about long wait times for pathology. More support required in psychosocial adjustments to 'successes' and 'failures' of treatments and clinical trials. Rationalization of side effects in light of the 'end-goal'.

1 BRAF: human gene encoding B-Raf protein.

Table 10.6 Final phase of the patient journey: A comparison of thematic findings from two data sources

Project A: 'Adaptation'		*Project B: 'Post-treatment and recurrence'*	
Health management related to surgery and medication	Organization of lifestyle around management of pain and discomfort of lymphoedema e.g., pumping out fluid each day and taking pump on vacation. Commitment to and appreciation of long-term relationships with healthcare providers involved in management of lymphoedema. Scheduling each day around large amounts of medication. Ongoing side effects of medication.	Long-term physical consequences	Managing change in lifestyle because of pain and discomfort of lymphoedema and other consequences such as severe peripheral neuropathy. Ongoing side effects of medication. Rationalizing long-term side effects and consequences of surgery and medication against positive outcome of survival.
Disease surveillance and psychosocial management of potential recurrence	Making personal commitment to regular scans regardless of logistical issues. Planning vacations and life events around timing of scans. Commitment to and appreciation of long-term relationship with oncologist and other healthcare providers involved in surveillance. Constant negotiation of feelings about high risk of recurrence.	Ongoing check-ups	Acknowledgement of lifelong dependence on healthcare for evidence of health. Acknowledgement of lifelong need for support to manage anxiety about recurrence and metastases. Unrequited expectations that clinicians in follow-up consultations will deal with psychosocial issues relating to fear of recurrence.
Dependence on healthcare services for personal life decisions	Vacation periods, cosmetic surgeries and permanent 'adornments' such as tattoos must be negotiated with oncologist.	Recurrence and metastases: the journey begins again	Symptoms less often skin-related and include lumps, pain, headaches, mobility issues and organ function impairment.

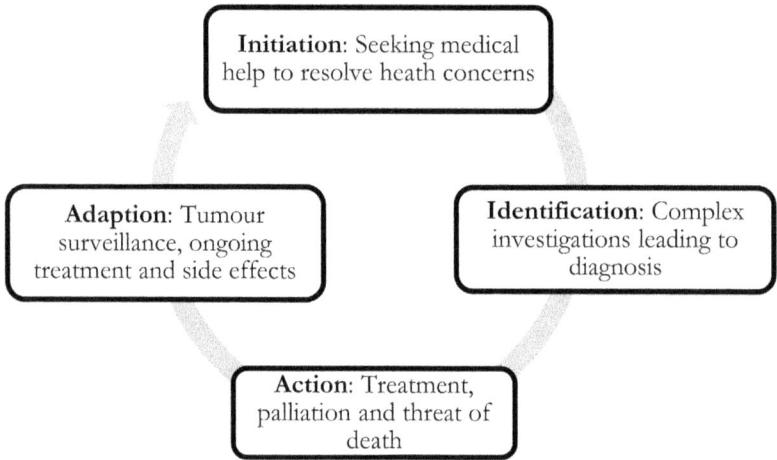

Figure 10.2 The circular plot of the clinical trajectory experienced by people with advanced and metastasized melanoma.

Source: Lamprell, K, M Chin, and J Braithwaite. 2019. ""Can I still get a tattoo?" Patients' experiences across the clinical trajectory for metastatic melanoma: A dynamic narrative model of patient journey." *Patient Experience Journal* 6 (1):87–93. https://pxjournal.org/journal/vol6/iss1/11

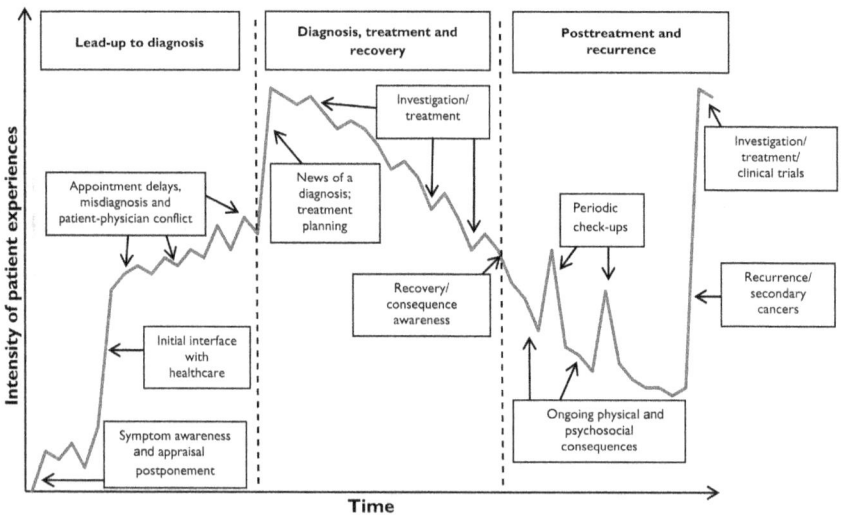

Figure 10.3 The meta-narrative plot of the clinical trajectory experienced by a general population of people with melanoma.

Source: Lamprell, K, and J Braithwaite. 2018. "When patients tell their own stories: A meta-narrative study of web-based personalized texts of 214 melanoma patients' journeys in four countries." *Qualitative Health Research* 28 (10):1564–1583, copyright © 2018 by SAGE Publications. Reprinted by Permission of SAGE Publications, Inc.

The plot model that resulted from the online ethnography was substantially linear and represented the peaks and troughs of the tensions wrought by healthcare experiences on the overall movement towards survival (Figure 10.3). Similarly to Figure 10.2, this plot accounts for transitions between phases of patient experience comprising grouped sets of clinical events, however this plot also comprises more detail through the representation of sub-sets of events and experiences.

The differences between the models may be explained by two key factors: 1) the specificity of the patient population in the lived ethnography, which comprised predominantly older, very ill people who had experienced one if not more cycles of patient journey for melanoma, and 2) the agency of the researcher in direct contact with the participant group from the lived ethnography research project but not with the authors of the online stories.

Conclusion

Clearly, nothing so neat and tidy as a model can represent the phenomenological nature of patients' experiences and we don't presume to have identified definitive narrative plots of the lived melanoma patient journey. However, we do see from this hybrid mode of inquiry the power of qualitative exploration to address the methodological gap between paradigmatic and whole-story investigations of patients' experiences of healthcare. This approach is important for further research into patient experience in general.

One additional aspect of our work has implications for longitudinal qualitative research. The use of ethnographic techniques to explore online environments is of increasing interest to social science researchers, largely because of the importance such spaces play in everyday life. Online environments provide places for people to connect with others and share experiences on a global scale. Their rich descriptions in online fora provide resource-efficient opportunities for qualitative researchers to examine patient journeys. Online narrative accounts offered us a data set complete with the collective, narratively framed longitudinal healthcare experiences of people with melanoma. When complemented by the data set from lived ethnography, we had an opportunity to understand the overarching plots of the melanoma journey from differing sets of patient perspectives.

To build resilience in managing the acute and then chronic system-wide burden of melanoma, healthcare organizations can benefit from a conceptualization of their role in these overarching narratives. Armed with knowledge of the sets of events that are of greater and lesser significance across patients' longitudinal journeys, healthcare organizations can be proactive in providing adequate resources of staff, patient information and supportive care services.

As Marie-Laure Ryan comments, "Nobody would walk into a book store and ask for a narrative" (2004, 6). Patients tell stories; researchers invest in their stories and extricate their stories from expansive, narrative data. We demonstrated the adaptability of qualitative healthcare methodologies in conjoining paradigmatic and narrative modes of inquiry, which are conventionally understood as disparate cognitions. The accomplishment – and the joy – of this work, was to produce meaningful findings for an audience of healthcare professionals, and current and future patients, from the generously shared stories of patients' journeys told by people with melanoma. We thank our participants for their time, and for the privilege of bearing witness to their transitions through the disruptions of illness and the world of patienthood.

References

Apalla, Z, A Lallas, E Sotiriou, E Lazaridou, and D Ioannides. 2017. "Epidemiological trends in skin cancer." *Dermatology Practical & Conceptual* 7 (2):1.

Ben-Tovim, DI, ML Dougherty, TJ O'Connell, and KM McGrath. 2008. "Patient journeys: The process of clinical redesign." *Medical Journal of Australia* 188 (S6):S14–S17.

Braithwaite, J. 2018. "Changing how we think about healthcare improvement." *BMJ* 361 (k2014).

Braithwaite, J, RL Wears, and E Hollnagel. 2015. "Resilient health care: Turning patient safety on its head." *International Journal for Quality in Health Care* 27 (5):418–420.

Braun, V, V Clarke, and N Rance. 2014. "How to use thematic analysis with interview data." In *The Counselling & Psychotherapy Research Handbook*, edited by A Vosserland and N Moller. London: Sage. 183–197.

Bruner, JS. 1986. *Actual Minds, Possible Worlds*. Cambridge: Harvard University Press.

Calman, L, L Brunton, and A Molassiotis. 2013. "Developing longitudinal qualitative designs: Lessons learned and recommendations for health services research." *BMC Medical Research Methodology* 13 (1):14.

Charon, R. 2008. *Narrative Medicine: Honoring the Stories of Illness*. New York: Oxford University Press.

Chattopadhyay, C, DW Kim, DS Gombos, J Oba, Y Qin, MD Williams, . . . SE Woodman. 2016. "Uveal melanoma: From diagnosis to treatment and the science in between." *Cancer* 122 (15):2299–2312.

Connelly, FM, and DJ Clandinin. 1990. "Stories of experience and narrative inquiry." *Educational Researcher* 19 (5):2–14.

Cornish, D, C Holterhues, LV Van de Poll-Franse, JW Coebergh, and T Nijsten. 2009. "A systematic review of health-related quality of life in cutaneous melanoma." *Annals of Oncology* 20 (S6):vi51–vi58.

Frank, AW. 2012. "Practicing dialogical narrative analysis." In *Varieties of Narrative Analysis*, edited by JA Holstein and JF Gubrium. Thousand Oaks: Sage.

Frank, AW. 2013. *The Wounded Storyteller: Body, Illness, and Ethics*. 2nd ed. Chicago: University of Chicago Press.

Grossoehme, D, and E Lipstein. 2016. "Analyzing longitudinal qualitative data: The application of trajectory and recurrent cross-sectional approaches." *BMC Research Notes* 9 (1):136.

Hill, DS, NDP Robinson, MP Caley, M Chen, EA O'Toole, JL Armstrong, . . . PE Lovat. 2015. "A novel fully humanized 3D skin equivalent to model early melanoma invasion." *Molecular Cancer Therapeutics* 14 (11):2665–2673.

Holland, J, R Thomson, and S Henderson. 2006. "Qualitative longitudinal research: A discussion paper." In *Families and Social Capital Working Papers*. London: South Bank University.

Hurwitz, B, and R Charon. 2013. "A narrative future for health care." *The Lancet* 381 (9881):1886–1887.

Ingold, T. 2011. *Being Alive: Essays on Movement, Knowledge and Description*. London: Routledge.

Lamprell, K, and J Braithwaite. 2016. "Patients as story-tellers of healthcare journeys." *Medical Humanities* 42 (3):207–209.

Lamprell, K, and J Braithwaite. 2018. "When patients tell their own stories: A meta-narrative study of web-based personalized texts of 214 melanoma patients' journeys in four countries." *Qualitative Health Research* 28 (10):1564–1583.

Lamprell, K, and J Braithwaite. 2019. "Reading between the lines: A five-point narrative approach to online accounts of illness." *Journal of Medical Humanities* 40 (4):569–590.

Lamprell, K, M Chin, and J Braithwaite. 2019. ""Can I still get a tattoo?" Patients' experiences across the clinical trajectory for metastatic melanoma: A dynamic narrative model of patient journey." *Patient Experience Journal* 6 (1):87–93.

Mattingly, C. 1998. *Healing Dramas and Clinical Plots: The Narrative Structure of Experience*. Cambridge: Cambridge University Press.

McLoone, J, K Watts, S Menzies, B Meiser, P Butow, and N Kasparian. 2013. "When the risks are high: Psychological adjustment among melanoma survivors at high risk of developing new primary disease." *Qualitative Health Research* 22 (8):1102–1113.

Miller, KD, RL Siegel, CC Lin, AB Mariotto, JL Kramer, JH Rowland, . . . A Jemal. 2016. "Cancer treatment and survivorship statistics." *CA: A Cancer Journal for Clinicians* 66 (4):271–289.

Palesh, O, A Aldridge-Gerry, K Bugos, D Pickham, J Chen, R Greco, and SM Swetter. 2014. "Health behaviors and needs of melanoma survivors." *Supportive Care in Cancer* 22 (11):2973–2980.

Panther, D, and DG Brodland. 2019. "Invasive melanoma." In *Evidence-Based Procedural Dermatology*, edited by A Murad. 2nd ed. New York: Springer International Publishing.

Polkinghorne, DE. 1995. "Narrative configuration in qualitative analysis: Narrative as story." *International Journal of Qualitative Studies in Education* 8 (1):5–23.

Ryan, M-L. 2004. *Narrative Across Media: The Languages of Storytelling*. Lincoln: University of Nebraska Press.

Smith, B, and AC Sparkes. 2008. "Changing bodies, changing narratives and the consequences of tellability: A case study of becoming disabled through sport." *Sociology of Health & Illness* 30 (2):217–236.

Thompson, JF, RA Scolyer, and RF Kefford. 2005. "Cutaneous melanoma." *The Lancet* 365 (9460):687–701.

Thomson, R, and J McLeod. 2015. "New frontiers in qualitative longitudinal research: An agenda for research." *International Journal of Social Research Methodology* 18 (3):243–250.

Trotter, SC, N Sroa, RR Winkelmann, T Olencki, and M Bechtel. 2013. "A global review of melanoma follow-up guidelines." *The Journal of Clinical and Aesthetic Dermatology* 6 (9):18.

Tsianakas, V, J Maben, T Wiseman, G Robert, A Richardson, P Madden, . . . EA Davies. 2012. "Using patients' experiences to identify priorities for quality improvement in breast cancer care: Patient narratives, surveys or both?" *BMC Health Services Research* 12 (1):271.

Walter, FM, L Birt, D Cavers, S Scott, J Emery, N Burrows, . . . C Campbell. 2014. "'This isn't what mine looked like': A qualitative study of symptom appraisal and help seeking in people recently diagnosed with melanoma." *BMJ Open* 4 (7):e005566.

Wears, R, E Hollnagel, and J Braithwaite. 2015. *Resilient Health Care: The Resilience of Everyday Clinical Work*. Vol. 2. Farnham: Ashgate Publishing, Ltd.

White, H. 1980. "The value of narrativity in the representation of reality." *Critical Inquiry* 7 (1):5–27.

11 Look the other way

Patient-centred care begins with care for our physicians. A dialogic narrative analysis of three personal essays

Klay Lamprell, Frances Rapport and Jeffrey Braithwaite

Introduction

Although patients are rightfully the focus of care, the needs of physicians and allied healthcare professionals can easily be ignored. Burnout now affects a third to a half of all clinicians at some point during their traineeships and careers (West, Dyrbye, and Shanafelt 2018; Rothenberger 2017; Rotenstein et al. 2016) and is characterized as having reached epidemic levels (West et al. 2016). Almost a third of 'residents' (or new doctors) will experience depression while undertaking their residencies (Mata et al. 2015), and binge-drinking affects over 40 per cent of doctors (Medisauskaite and Kamau 2019; West et al. 2009).

The crisis for doctors is long-standing and well known. The research literature reflects decades of quantitative and qualitative work investigating the extent to which doctors suffer and why. More recently, evidence is also emerging of the associations between clinician safety ratings and emotional exhaustion, depersonalization and personal accomplishment (Welp, Meier, and Manser 2015). In response, initiatives to address stress and promote physician well-being are becoming more common. The reality, however, is that some key contributing factors to physician suffering, particularly economic and political pressures, are not readily solved and indeed are intensifying (Braithwaite 2018).

Against this backdrop and given the wealth of empirical knowledge about physician burnout, we need to consider what future direction research can take in investigating this 'sorry state of affairs'. For our interests in this book in particular we need to understand how qualitative methodology might make a contribution. Here we propose a shift in qualitative perspective. Rather than seeking patterns and commonality across populations of physicians by interpreting singular experiences as instances of the universal, we explored engagement with the singularity of doctors' stories of burnout.

Doctors are prolific writers. In part this is because physicians bear witness to, and have a role to play in, the drama of lives ruptured by illness. In part it is because the practice of medicine is a narrative endeavour (Charon 2008) – science practiced through the receiving and telling of stories, in interactions with patients and in conversations with other healthcare providers. Finally, it is because the narrative endeavour of medical practice engages with a fundamental human need – for wellness – and the complex relationship humans have with their bodies (Johna and Rahman 2011). It is no wonder then that when physicians "have faced their most human limitations" (Wilson, Millard, and Sabroe 2019, 21) they write about it.

Through their books, blogs and online narrative essays, physicians are inviting audiences into imaginative spaces that reconstruct the events and outcomes of burnout – the physical and emotional exhaustion, the feelings of depersonalization and the sense of diminished personal accomplishment (West, Dyrbye, and Shanafelt 2018). In the telling of their stories, the deep disruptions to personal and professional identity, and perhaps also the reclaiming of self, can be witnessed.

This chapter situates doctors' autobiographical texts – online narrative essays about experiences of burnout in particular – as fields of close qualitative inquiry. Online narratives are a fast-emerging source of qualitative data on personal experience (Lamprell and Braithwaite 2018; Wilson, Kenny, and Dickson-Swift 2015) and are increasingly valued as a significant contribution to the evolution of qualitative methods of research (Redlich-Amirav and Higginbottom 2014). To our knowledge, however, physicians' online narrative essays have not yet featured in qualitative research on physician stress and burnout.

We explore three personal accounts using a dialogic analysis, which is also known as performative analysis. This approach concentrates on narrative as dialogue and the ways that it assembles, performs, transmits and interacts with "personal and cultural realities" (Smith et al. 2009, 343) relative to others. The focus is on the dimensions of narrative that develop the "orientation of discourse" (Bakhtin 1983, 279) such as genre; the embedding of professional, personal, ideological views; the "authorial intentions" (Bakhtin 1983, 324); and the stakes "riding on telling this story, at this time, to these listeners" (Frank 2012a, 33).

Background on physician burnout

Increasing patient workload, high staffing turnover, the time-consuming management of electronic health records (Shanafelt et al. 2016; Gawante 2018), medico-legal constraints, the imperatives of patient-centred performance metrics, attendance to top-down workplace policies (Montgomery 2014; Mintzberg 1992) as well as obligations to play formal and informal leadership roles (Denis and van Gestel 2016) are amongst a number of factors putting pressure on healthcare professionals.

These pressures add to the inherent challenges of healthcare settings, which can be "hectic, demanding, time-constrained environments" (Rivera-Rodriguez and Karsh 2010, 304) in which there may be lack of control over – and poor capacity to plan for – patients' situations and needs. Additionally, temperament and personality profiling of clinicians suggests they may be conscientious to an extreme level (Peters and King 2012) and may put themselves under pressure by being obsessional in their execution of their work (Akiskal, Savino, and Akiskal 2005).

Physician burnout is then a complex, multifaceted issue with no easy 'fix'. Calls for initiatives to support doctors in managing pressures and reducing anxiety are becoming more insistent (Dyrbye et al. 2017; Davis et al. 2003). In response, educational institutions and healthcare organizations are devising and implementing varied programs and interventions (Shanafelt, Dyrbye, and West 2017, 902), most of which are individually-focused or aimed at achieving local results (Montgomery 2014).

These programs include cognitive-behavioural, relaxation and mindfulness training for groups of doctors (Clough et al. 2017; Ireland et al. 2017) and collaborative activities such as Schwarz rounds, which are multidisciplinary forums in which "healthcare staff within an organization discuss the psychological, emotional and social challenges associated with their work in a confidential and safe environment" (Robert et al. 2017, 1). The success of such programs is often hampered, ironically, by lack of funding to cover doctors for participation during the workday (West et al. 2016).

Emerging organization-wide initiatives include modifications to clinical work processes, such as shortened clinical rotations (Mikkelsen et al. 2019), reduced resident shifts (West et al. 2016) and the use of scribes who support physician workflow by documenting patient encounters in real time and entering data in electronic medical records (Gidwani et al. 2017). The cacophony of physicians' voices weighing in on this issue, with narrative accounts of burnout and expert opinions on how to frame and label the crisis, point to frustration with the lack of overarching resolution. We turn now to some examples from those narratives.

Methodology

Our intention was not to theorize the phenomenon of burnout amongst physicians but to witness the singular, narrative perspectives that are missing from empirical work to date. 'Narrative' resists definition and is perhaps best explained by description. In narrative, says Arthur Frank, "lives come from somewhere and are going somewhere" (Frank 2002, 5). Narratives, explains Catherine Kohler Riessman, take a listener into a world of consequential events, often exposing a "breach between ideal and real, self and society" (Riessman 1993, 3).

"Narrative analysis takes as its objective of investigation the story itself" (Riessman 1993, 1). Riessman identifies three key approaches to narrative analysis that may be used independently of each other or together: thematic, structural and dialogic/performative (Riessman 2008). The thematic approach is concerned with thematizing events and topics which become apparent to the analyst via the content. The structural approach attends to the structure and use of language and textual sequencing to organize the telling of events and the communication of topics. The dialogic/performative approach may consider the thematic nature of the content and the structural means by which content is organized, but is chiefly concerned with "who an utterance may be directed to, when, and why, that is, for what purposes?" (Riessman 2008, 105).

We adopted the dialogic/performative approach here because it is suited to understanding deconstruction, reconstruction and ambiguity of personal identity framed by social and cultural conditions and pressures (Riessman 1993). Rita Charon (2008) affirms the relevance of the process to our project's intentions when she asks, "For where more than in the medical context, so rife with power inequities and rigid hierarchies, does one need to call out our social embeddedness and contingent identities?" (Charon et al. 2016, 86).

Text choice

Looking for personal perspective essays, we scoped English-language health websites and blogs focused on health and medicine and reviewed medical journals. We used the primary search term 'burnout' (or 'physician burnout') and the secondary terms 'wellness' (or 'physician wellness'), 'depression' (or 'physician depression') and 'stress' (or 'physician stress'). We continued the search until the point of saturation. The search was conducted over a period of eight months, from August 2018 to March 2019.

Texts identified as relevant were briefly reviewed by the primary researcher [KL] to differentiate content that was narrative in its account of personal experience from content offering expert opinion reflecting empirical research. This was a deeply iterative process. Essays offering expert opinions often used an experiential opening paragraph describing a personal experience of burnout, which threw up a number of 'false positives'. Additionally, texts commonly contained internal links to other texts published on the same website or links to external websites, with some posts published to multiple websites.

With this high level of snowballing and the repetitive readings of same or similar texts on different websites, the scoping process was often obfuscating. Though we initially maintained a register of information tracking our search – such as may be relevant to a PRISMA search representation in a systematic review – we eventually understood the iterative nature of this search and the fluid nature of the Internet as a publishing medium to render this an ultimately impracticable endeavour. As an indication of the scope, our search took us to numerous sites and journals with bases located in Australia, New Zealand, the United States, Canada and the United Kingdom and we read over 400 texts of some 700 to 1,000 words per text.

The methodology of dialogic/performative analysis does not seek to identify patterns or commonalities across multiple stories, so it does not rely for its substance and outcome on analysis of a large number of texts. Indeed, its intention of 'close reading' (Charon 2008) demands that a research report either dispense with word limits or, as in our circumstance, limit the number of texts that are analyzed.

Frank notes that "most qualitative methodologists would, at this point, recommend some systematic method for sorting through the stories that have been collected and making accountable decisions about which ones the analysis will focus on; their sense of method lies in that accountability" (Frank 2012a, 43). Frank identifies that – in contrast to this process of accountability – dialogic/performative analysis commits to the unique interpretive choices of the researcher during analysis. Following Aristotle's *Nicomachean Ethics* (Ross 1925) which allows for researcher *phronesis* (Frank 2012a; Flyvbjerg 2001) – a practical wisdom – Frank situates experienced researchers as intuitive 'spotters' of valuable stories. He finds that this kind of practical wisdom "can never be fully articulated . . . but is felt as a guiding force" (Frank 2012b, 57).

We selected three texts for analysis (Ahronheim 2019; Moulder 2018; Topin 2018). Our choices were shaped by epistemological commitments to the singularity of experiences and by the value to the research report of presenting three totally different kinds of texts, each speaking to different audiences and each reflecting different experiences of burnout.

Procedures

Dialogism as explored and interpreted by Bakhtin (1983), Riessman (1993), Charon (2008), Charon et al. (2016) and Frank (2012a) provided us with an overall understanding of dialogic/performative analysis. In our approach to each text we were guided by Frank's key concepts in dialogic analysis (see Box 11.1). In undertaking the analysis of each text, we used Frank's five key prompts (Frank 2012a): resources, circulation, affiliation, identity and stakes. We have interpreted each of these prompts in Table 11.1. We formatted our reporting of our analysis to parallel this suite of prompts tabled.

Box 11.1   Ethical position or ontology in dialogic/ performative analysis, adapted from Frank (2012a)

The researcher's practice of dialogic/performative analysis:

- Keeps up a tension between the researcher's personal relationality to the text and the analysis of the text. To this end, Charon proposes that "in all contexts we call upon our analytic skills while remaining attentive to our affective responses to the texts and to one another" (Charon et al. 2016, 119).
- Understands that dialogic/performative analysis is uniquely interpretive and the value of its conclusions depend on creative attention to method, not on reproducibility of outcomes.
- Values witnessing and describing the life worlds of narrative accounts as an effective contribution to qualitative social science. Viewed another way, this form of analysis does not presuppose that "humans are not organizing some aspect of their lives as well as they could" (Frank 2012a, 38) making it necessary to propose solutions through the findings of the research.
- Proceeds from interest in a story's standpoint of personal troubles (Frank 2000) taking into account that storytellers make choices to privilege certain aspects of their experiences in order to "report their reality as they need to tell it as well as reporting what they believe their listeners are prepared to hear" (Frank 2012a, 38).
- Acknowledges that the research report conveys – perhaps highlights – a reality already told by the storyteller and is not exposing some reality of which the author herself or himself did not conceive.

Table 11.1 Analytic prompts for dialogic/performative research

Prompt	Framed as question	Examples
Resources	What narrative means or devices does the story use to represent experience and how could it be different if it used different resources?	Stories already circulating; recognizable character types, plot lines, grand narratives, genre choices and tropes.
Circulation	Who tells which stories to whom? How is the story framed to anticipate certain readers (or publication)? Who might object to a story?	Publishing communities; communities of practice as self-enclosed storytelling groups.
Affiliation	What boundaries does the story set for who will affiliate with its telling and who might be excluded from the 'we' who share the story?	Political and cultural constraints, and allegiances.
Identity	How do people tell stories to explore who they might become and how does the story teach people (storyteller and audience) who they are?	Unique representations; stereotypes; allowances for ambiguity and unfinalized identities; preferences for finalized rendering.
Stakes	What does the act of storytelling put at stake for the storyteller and audience – what vulnerabilities does its telling and its receiving expose?	Individual storytellers with human frailties.

Analysis

Story 1: 'It can be exhausting to care': A letter to all new junior doctors

Precis: This is the story of an orthopedic surgeon, speaking to junior doctors to let them know that she understands and can relate to how burnt out they might be feeling at this stage of their careers. She portrays the physical, emotional and intellectual disturbances they may be experiencing – the inadequate sleep, the grab-and-go diet, the ongoing worry about patients and the concern about their suitability to the job. She then describes the shift that will occur over time and how they will grow into their identities as doctors and find meaning in their work.

Story 2: On the other side of physician burnout

Precis: This story tells us of a pulmonary and critical care physician who burnt out incrementally over more than a decade. Multiple workplace and personal factors contributed ultimately to an exhaustion and a trepidation about work that he couldn't resolve. His ensuing identity crisis compelled him to reconsider the way his life was set up and to make provision for the priorities of mental health and family life.

Table 11.2 Story 1 dialogic/performative analysis

Resources	The storyteller chooses to call her essay a letter and employs the conventions of that genre by opening the essay with the dialogic pronouns 'you' and 'we': "The job of a junior doctor isn't what you thought it would be". A click on the storyteller's name reveals our 'letter-writer' is an orthopedic surgeon, so the letter can be understood as a form of mentorship.
Circulation	The story is published on the online international edition of *The Guardian* which is an independently owned newspaper based in the United Kingdom. It was published in the 'Blood, sweat and tears' segment of the newspaper, which is described as featuring "healthcare professionals' accounts of moments in their career that have been joyous, life-changing, difficult or just plain awful". The essay was therefore generally intended to reach a readership of healthcare professionals or those interested in personal accounts of healthcare professionals, and, given its title, in particular junior doctors. Physicians 'burnout' has been discussed in the media as a controversial schema, (Oliver 2017) a victimizing or blaming characterization suggestive of a lack of personal resilience or willingness to work hard. For junior doctors aiming to show they have what it takes, the label of burnout is a threat. The storyteller stays away from the use of that word and refers instead to one of the key indicators – exhaustion. In this way she is sure not to repel the very readers she hopes to attract.
Affiliation	The intention made explicit by the title is affiliation with junior doctors. The tool of affiliation is the convention of letter-writing. Confident of her solidarity with her assumed readership, she describes the experiences they are going through: "You are losing weight . . .". She tells them she knows this is because they don't have time to eat lunch, that their to-do list grows faster than they can complete tasks and they are constantly called on their bleep if they leave the ward to go to the canteen.
	To ensure affinity with the widest audience of junior doctors, the narrator broadens the range of the experiences she is describing: "Or maybe you are gaining weight . . .". Again, she details why this is happening. 'You', she says, don't have the capacity to prepare food and plan for healthy eating, and end up eating from the vending machine or living off the doughnuts at the nursing station.
	The key point of dialogic kinship, summed up in the title, is that caring for self too little and caring for others too much is a critical juncture for junior doctors: "You lie in bed", she says, and think of sick patients and then get up at 3am to phone the night shift doctor or nurses to check those patients are okay. She knows that 'you' are wondering if you care too much. "You can't switch off; this does not feel sustainable".
	The junior doctor's experience of this level of caring, she understands, is lonely and apocalyptic. It can feel that there is no value in your services, or worse, that your lack of experience and slowness are making things more difficult for other doctors, and worse still, 'you' can feel that "you're not cut out to be a doctor". This is the climax in her characterization of shared experience, a point at which no more need be said about the hardship. Now the narrator turns 'you' to look at a different perspective, one that contradicts your sense of loneliness and unequivocally brings 'you' into the secret folds of your professional community: "Every doctor has felt like this. Every doctor has pretended not to feel like this".

(*Continued*)

Table 11.2 (Continued)

Identity	Letting junior doctors know that all others before them have felt as unsure and as isolated as they now feel is a linkage, a lifeline, a social tie that each junior doctor can grasp at to assure themselves of their worth as physicians. The sentence shifts the text into a united telling of experience. The personal pronoun becomes 'we'. And with 'we' comes relief – the comfort of causality between temporal progression and wisdom gained as communal professional identity is established: "Over time we have learned . . . to look after ourselves first. The routine tasks become easier, and we improve at time management and prioritization. We learn to hand over to the next team, another person, or the next day".
	Having offered her 'fledglings' the lifeline of knowledge that the visceral sensitivity of inexperience will pass, she makes a plea to their still developing and vulnerable professional identities. She asks them to "please keep on caring". She characterizes how that caring identity will 'look': "We have slowly accepted that being a doctor is not about helping people, but caring for them", which, she says, can be an exhausting and thankless task. Patients don't want to hear that they have to stop smoking, have more blood tests, subject themselves to intimidating procedures like nasogastric tubing. "The rewards are not gratification . . . the satisfaction has to come from within".
Stakes	This balance of caring for self and for others, this challenge of finding satisfaction within, is what the narrator believes is at stake for these doctors. Those stakes, she suggests, can be moderated by finding the work that has the most synergy with their desires and values. She tells them that a medical degree opens the door to a range of specialties so "you will find the job that suits you".
	In reaching out to junior doctors in this way, she reaches within. She must have lived all this to be able to tell it. The stakes of caring for herself also must have been high, must have taken their toll. Otherwise she could not know what it feels like when reality sets in.

Table 11.3 Story 2 dialogic/performative analysis

Resources	In the opening sentence the narrator contrasts the story to come with that of a television doctor. He makes use of the readers' assumed familiarity with popular medical dramas to establish an accessible contrast with his real world experience. "I've watched enough television shows to know what a burned-out physician is supposed to look like: crying in the stairwell, head hanging dejectedly, knees bent; the downward spiral into drugs and alcohol that leads to a near-miss in surgery; or the final, explosive monologue that alienates the doctor in front of patients and peers. A once-solid doctor now broken . . .". And then we learn, "Mine didn't happen that way".
	He draws his readers into the imaginative space of his burnout with an accessible trope – the activity of a stalagmite in the making, compounding its deposits of competing obligations:
	"*Drip*: Twelve years of hustling at a hectic pace in a private pulmonary and critical care practice . . .
	Drip: The never-ending clicks to provide documentation in the electronic medical record . . .

	Drip: The frivolous suit I was dragged into by virtue of having been on call for the hospital one night. . .
	Drip: . . . Trying to be actively engaged in the lives of my wife and children with half my brain still in the hospital and the other half fighting the weight of cumulative fatigue".
Circulation	The essay is published on STAT news which is a health-oriented news website launched on 4 November 2015. It is produced by Boston Globe Media. The essay was published on its 'First Opinion' segment which features perspectives and opinions on medicine, biotechnology and the life sciences. The site speaks to a wide community of practitioners involved in healthcare and medical-related sciences however the title declares that this is about a physician's experience. This is the essay's only endeavour to focus the readership. The end of the article notes that the author is a part-time pulmonary and critical care physician which may serve to further filter the audience interest.
	As noted in the previous essay, the 'burnout' label can be contentious, however the title of this essay renders it 'benign' – the burnout is now over and readers need not consider how they should weigh in on the accuracy of the label. The end of the essay notes that an earlier version of the article appeared on the author's blog, suggesting the author is dedicated to circulating his story to the widest possible audience.
Affiliation	The key affiliations developed in this essay between reader and narrator lie in the narrator's candid sharing of his identity transformation. He makes no special effort to assign relational elements to his story, though when he tells us about the approach he took to resolve his burnout, he is explicit about his dialogic intention: he wants us to know that he has no aspiration to the mantle of champion burnout survivor. "This approach certainly won't work for all physicians who are burned out. But it's working for me".
Identity	The narrator prepares us early for the identity transformation to come, heralding that he did not see himself as a typical burnout candidate, and then taking us through his symptoms and onto his outcome. In describing the transformation, his identity as narrator undergoes shifts. The poised comparison of self with the fictional television doctor and the poetic voice of the stalagmite analogy is an effort that seems to exhaust the narrator. He suddenly departs from the subjective dimensions of his narrative and tells us the facts of his experience as they might be understood in a guidebook on burnout: "A physician's slow burn is often masked by his or her defense mechanisms and denial. But it eventually becomes apparent . . . when the excitement and potential of each new morning is replaced by the dread of what might lie ahead . . . when it feels as though patients and staff are no longer expressing themselves but are instead complaining and whining".
	Yet the need to find refuge in impersonality is temporary; he quickly returns to the 'I' of the story and describes the symptoms of burnout that he manifested: "I found myself becoming exhausted at work. I became more callous, impatient, and terse with my patients. With residents, medical students, nurses, and my physician partners. With friends. And with my family".

(Continued)

Table 11.3 (Continued)

	Awareness of this different version of himself prompted him to seek change – change he hoped he could define in terms of obvious "fixable, external" problems like staff shortages and time spent on electronic medical records. The alternative, he tells us, was to look within, which was frightening: "Because if those weren't the cause of my problem, maybe I needed to look at myself. Was I too weak? Did I not have enough fortitude, endurance, or grit? With those thoughts of weakness came feelings of shame".
	'Weakness' and 'shame', he explains, have played no part in his experience of life. "I've completed six Ironman triathlons. I'm a water polo goalie . . . I survived four years of medical school and four years as a resident in internal medicine and pediatrics".
	Yet he felt he was no longer capable of "taking challenges head on".
	He made changes, deciding to work part-time, and is still coming to terms with his new sense of self. "Did I fail? I don't think so, but that's something I am still processing". Freed from a paradigm of opposing identities – strong or weak, resilient or needy, solid or broken – he is learning a new way to be a physician. "I am not broken" he says. "I am just getting started".
Stakes	The narrator's first thoughts were to leave the profession entirely, to reorient his professional identity and become a science school teacher, or find other ways to use his training and his skills. His life with his family was at stake, and he needed "the emotional and physical energy to be patient and present, not irritable and dismissive". He thought "about patients who had made a tremendous impact on my life, of decisions made and opportunities missed".
	He explains now that he writes to us down the track from that decision to work part-time, with the stakes of that decision still high: "I sold my partnership and with it my safety net . . . I am still getting used to it. There's more time but far less income . . . financial choices are harder and retirement less certain. There's more freedom, but maybe not enough structure". Risks remain, but the coda in his description of what those risks allow indicates that he has time now to be a parent, to be a student, to coach water polo, to train as a triathlete, to be a husband and, as a part-time doctor, to re-embrace "the challenge and privilege of taking care of patients when they are at their sickest and most vulnerable".

Story 3: Please, be kind to your doctor. We need it.

Precis: This is a story of an emergency physician who is grappling with exhaustion from overwork and struggling with heightened emotionality. She explains that while she feels burnt out, she isn't comfortable with the word 'burnout' because it fails to describe the complexity of her feelings and her situation. She prefers to work with the action-oriented idea of 'wellness', and as a first step towards wellness, she asks for help from her readers. We can help by taking her humanity into account when we interact with her, by considering the effort it takes to care for each patient and the time she spends away from her own family in order to attend to our needs. She wants us to see our interaction with her – and other doctors – as a relationship in which we each care for the other.

Table 11.4 Story 3 dialogic/performative analysis

Resources	If there is a genre of online narrative essay, it borrows from published journals and memoirs. Its voice is dialogic and intimate, so we are comfortable with the opening paragraph in which this narrator speaks to us as confidants. "There's always so much to write about, and there's never any time. I work too much; it's become evident recently that I need to cut down". What she goes on to say, however, is surprising if not shocking: "There are days I hide my tears, and days I show my tears, when before the tears would have waited for the occasional (yes, occasional) shower". A doctor who showers only occasionally defies the archetype. Like our previous author, she is now far removed from the character we idealize for our physicians. The storyteller is not constrained by narrative type-casting. She will continue to surprise us. The colloquial and familiar voice of her narrator – "Burnout. There, I said it again" – will soon become urgent as she begins an emotional plea for us to come to her aid. In this she will again confront our conceptions – doctors do not ask patients for help. The archetypes are challenged at every turn, perhaps reflecting the chaos of burnout.
Circulation	The story is published on the website www.kevinmd.com which characterizes itself as "social media's leading physician voice". It is a commercial website with 150,000 subscribers that is open to the public. Authors are responsible for the material they post. The essay had received six comments at the time of writing this chapter, 16 days after its posting to the site. The essay is posted in the section 'Physician' and by clicking through we find that the author is described as an emergency physician. The title is a direct appeal to patients and in the body of the essay she widens the appeal of her patient audience by referencing not only the emergency department, but the family doctor's office and specialists' clinics.
Affiliation	The title draws us immediately to the narrator's side: "Please, be kind to your doctor. We need it". We would be heartless to ignore her petition. The narrative she then takes us on is not a progression of external events but of her thoughts. Overtures of her exhaustion lead to a tussle with the label of burnout. In order to make an end to her discomfort with that characterization of herself, she must make a beginning elsewhere, and that beginning involves us. It requires that we affiliate with her circumstances. "How can you help? Can you help? Can anyone? I think so. Here's an idea. Next time you're in the emergency department, or your family doctor's office, or visiting a specialist in a clinic, try to think about how hard those individuals are working for your benefit". Her final entreaty comes full circle from the title. "So please, be kind to your doctor. We need it. We need kindness and compassion. From you, from each other, from ourselves".
Identity	Lack of time to write, to express all the things she wants to say, is declared upfront as a source of pain: she has no "me-time". The consequence is that "things affect me much more than they ever did. . . . This is a function of my level of exhaustion". She is, she feels, at the point of burnout, or on her way there. The idea of burnout links her with those who suffer in her professional community and moves her to shift from 'I' to 'we'.

(*Continued*)

Table 11.4 (Continued)

	Yet she struggles to lay claim to burnout: "A small word we use a lot recently, to describe a very complex situation". She includes herself as one of the many who "won't mention it, won't give it breath to solidify itself in our lives. If we say it, we make it real, when it's often easier to just push it away and deny its existence. . . . To be honest, I'm not always sure this is where I am; but I'd like to learn how to prevent getting there". As a contingency, she is willing to engage with another prevailing identity, that of 'physician wellbeing'. "This is something I can hang my hat on, that I want to be a part of". She then tells us that the absence of our compassion for her, and for her colleagues, is part of the problem. It is not an issue of power relations or diminished physician status but of identifying as humans sharing events of significance. Her plea is that we 'see' her, that we understand the sacrifices she and her colleagues are making, that we empathize with the ways in which their personal lives are impacted by the demands of their profession. "Put yourselves in our shoes, for a moment, and see through our eyes. See the way we have to hide our own emotions in order to help you get through yours. See how we stay late to take care of your children, while our own children miss us at home". Finally, she seats her personal well-being in the mutually intimate nature of the patient-doctor relationship. "Please, look at me and see my heart, see my humanity, treat me as you would like me to treat you, with kindness . . . I feel what you feel. I hurt as you hurt. I bring your stories and your pain home . . . I am changed, by you, and you by me. And it hurts". The narrator's identity and our own are inextricably linked.
Stakes	The stakes of labeling herself as burnt out are high enough to move this narrator quickly from idea to action. She surprises us when she addresses us directly to declare that one of the ideas for recovery involves us, and she does not let go of us; the essay shifts into focused intersubjectivity and steadily drills the need for us to share the dilemma of conflicting pressures on healthcare delivery. The risk of not responding to her is the quality of care we receive: "Look at all of us, stretched far beyond what we ever thought we signed up for, in a system where more and more sick people come to our door but we can't hire more physicians to help see all of you faster". Ultimately however, it is her story and her wellness that is at stake with the final plea: "Help us heal, the way we try to heal you".

Discussion

Though having suffered, these 'doctors as writers' are not victims. Amid the exact-ing descriptions in these essays of what we know empirically to be widely correct, we see that each of these doctors works hard through their writing to make con-nections with their intended readers and to seed shared experiences. Choosing to tell their stories within the structures of autobiographical narrative is an act that intentionally diverts from universal knowledge, inviting audiences to connect with the unique ways that burnout arrives into physicians' lives, the distinctive havoc it inflicts and the exceptional need for compassion it generates.

Narrative as an "instrument for self-knowledge and communion" (Charon et al. 2016, 139) allows these physicians to shape singular identities that are far removed from their roles as diagnosticians, detached scientists, income-maximizers and organizational operatives. Through close attention to the dialogic nature of these narratives we open up "continuing possibilities of listening and of responding to what is heard" (Frank 2012a, 37). The aim of dialogic analysis is not to summarize findings but to connect into the telling of the story, and to be conscious in our response.

Using the five key prompts, we reflect: the current environment of healthcare in which physicians can widely disseminate their stories; the types of medical practice that frame physicians' experiences; the audiences to whom physicians are 'speaking'; the aims of physicians in telling their story; and the consequences of telling that story in that particular way. Such analysis, Mark Bamberg suggests, is "invested in both the means and the way these means are put to use to arrive at presentations and interpretations of meaningful experiences" (Bamberg 2012, 2).

Future directions

Continuing to research the organizational factors that cause stress, depression and burnout in frontline healthcare professionals is simply more of the same. After decades of research, we know the factors. Some are amenable to being addressed – too few clinicians for the patient workload, fewer resources than are needed, detached management, a toxic culture, poor support structures, etc. Others are fundamental to the caring professions – the vulnerabilities of patients in need, the suffering of fellow humans, the necessity to inflict pain in order to attempt to help or cure. Healthcare professionals on the frontline of care know the factors. They know what it is about the system that is making them feel burnt out or unwell in other ways. They are narrating the magnitude of the professional obligation to make patients well – the relentless illness dramas of people's lives to which they are privy, from which they wish to learn and grow – despite organizational pressures and constraints. They are entrusting audiences with their own vulnerabilities.

Qualitative researchers can enter this dialogue to witness the commitment and passion of doctors and to acknowledge their suffering. The 'doctor-as-God' paradigm of healthcare is long gone, and patients are increasingly cared for in ways that respect their values and personal needs, but have we forgotten to care for our carers? We need to look both ways.

References

Ahronheim, S. 2019. "Please, be kind to your doctor. We need it." *KevinMD*, 10 June. Accessed 6 August 2019. www.kevinmd.com/blog/2019/06/please-be-kind-to-your-doctor-we-need-it.html.

Akiskal, K, M Savino, and H Akiskal. 2005. "Temperament profiles in physicians, lawyers, managers, industrialists, architects, journalists, and artists: A study in psychiatric outpatients." *Journal of Affective Disorders* 85 (1–2):201–206.

Bakhtin, M. 1983. *The Dialogic Imagination*. Austin: University of Texas Press.

Bamberg, M. 2012. "Narrative analysis." In *APA Handbook of Research Methods in Psychology*, edited by H Cooper, P Camic, D Long, A Panter, D Rindskopf, and K Sher. Washington, DC: American Psychological Association Press.

Braithwaite, J. 2018. "Changing how we think about healthcare improvement." *BMJ* 361 (k2014).

Charon, R. 2008. *Narrative Medicine: Honoring the Stories of Illness*. New York: Oxford University Press.

Charon, R, S DasGupta, N Hermann, ER Marcus, and M Spiegel. 2016. *The Principles and Practice of Narrative Medicine*. New York: Oxford University Press.

Clough, B, S March, R Chan, L Casey, R Phillips, and M Ireland. 2017. "Psychosocial interventions for managing occupational stress and burnout among medical doctors: A systematic review." *Systematic Reviews* 6 (1):144.

Davis, M, T Detre, D Ford, W Hansbroug, H Hendin, J Laszlo, . . . S Miles. 2003. "Confronting depression and suicide in physicians: A consensus statement." *JAMA* 289 (23):3161–3166.

Denis, J, and N van Gestel. 2016. "Medical doctors in healthcare leadership: Theoretical and practical challenges." *BMC Health Services Research* 16 (2):158.

Dyrbye, L, T Shanafelt, C Sinsky, P Cipriano, J Bhatt, A Ommaya, . . . D Meyers. 2017. Burnout among health care professionals: A call to explore and address this underrecognized threat to safe, high-quality care. *NAM Perspectives Discussion Paper*, Washington, DC.

Flyvbjerg, B. 2001. *Making Social Science Matter: Why Social Inquiry Fails and How It Can Succeed Again*. Translated by S Sampson. Cambridge: Cambridge University Press.

Frank, AW. 2000. "The standpoint of storyteller." *Qualitative Health Research* 10 (3):354–365.

Frank, AW. 2002. "Why study people's stories? The dialogical ethics of narrative analysis." *International Journal of Qualitative Methods* 1 (1).

Frank, AW. 2012a. "Practicing dialogical narrative analysis." In *Varieties of Narrative Analysis*, edited by JA Holstein and JF Gubrium. Thousand Oaks: Sage.

Frank, AW. 2012b. "Reflective healthcare practice: Claims, phronesis, and dialogue." In *Phronesis as Professional Knowledge: Implications for Education and Practice*, edited by E Kinsella and A Pitman. Rotterdam: Sense Publishers.

Gawante, A. 2018. "Why doctors hate their computers." *The New Yorker*, 5 November. Accessed 6 August 2019. www.newyorker.com/magazine/2018/11/12/why-doctors-hate-their-computers.

Gidwani, R, C Nguyen, A Kofoed, C Carragee, T Rydel, I Nelligen, . . . S Lin. 2017. "Impact of Scribes on Physician Satisfaction, Patient Satisfaction, and Charting Efficiency: A Randomized Controlled Trial." *Annals of Family Medicine* 15 (5):427–433.

Ireland, M, B Clough, K Gill, F Langan, A O'Connor, and L Spencer. 2017. "A randomized controlled trial of mindfulness to reduce stress and burnout among intern medical practitioners." *Medical Teacher* 39 (4):409–414.

Johna, S, and S Rahman. 2011. "Humanity before science: Narrative medicine, clinical practice, and medical education." *The Permanente Journal* 15 (4):92–94.

Lamprell, K, and J Braithwaite. 2018. "When patients tell their own stories: A meta-narrative study of web-based personalized texts of 214 melanoma patients' journeys in four countries." *Qualitative Health Research* 28 (10):1564–1583.

Mata, DA, MA Ramos, N Bansal, R Khan, C Guille, E Di Angelantonio, and S Sen. 2015. "Prevalence of depression and depressive symptoms among resident physicians: A systematic review and meta-analysis." *JAMA* 314 (22):2373–2383.

Medisauskaite, A, and C Kamau. 2019. "Does occupational distress raise the risk of alcohol abuse, binge-eating, ill health and sleep problems among medical doctors? A UK cross-sectional study." *BMJ Open* 9 (e027362).

Mikkelsen, ME, BJ Anderson, L Bellini, WD Schweickert, BD Fuchs, and MP Kerlin. 2019. "Burnout, and fulfillment, in the profession of critical care medicine." *American Journal of Respiratory and Critical Care Medicine*.

Mintzberg, H. 1992. *Structures in Fives: Designing Effective Organisations*. 1st ed. New York: Prentice Hall.

Montgomery, AA. 2014. "The inevitability of physician burnout: Implications for interventions." *Burnout Research* 1 (1):50–56.

Moulder, E. 2018. "'It can be exhausting to care': A letter to all new junior doctors." *The Guardian*, 18 October. Accessed 6 August 2019. www.theguardian.com/society/2018/oct/18/exhausting-care-letter-new-junior-doctors.

Oliver, D. 2017. "Challenging the victim narrative about NHS doctors." *BMJ* 359 (j4304).

Peters, M, and J King. 2012. "Perfectionism in doctors." *BMJ* 344:e1674.

Redlich-Amirav, D, and G Higginbottom. 2014. "New emerging technologies in qualitative research." *The Qualitative Report* 19 (26):1–14.

Riessman, CK. 1993. *Narrative Analysis. Vol. 30, Qualitative Methods*. Thousand Oaks: Sage.

Riessman, CK. 2008. *Narrative Methods for the Human Sciences*. Thousand Oaks: Sage.

Rivera-Rodriguez, A, and B Karsh. 2010. "Interruptions and distractions in healthcare: Review and reappraisal." *Quality & Safety in Health Care* 19 (4):304–312.

Robert, G, J Philippou, M Leamy, E Reynolds, S Ross, L Bennett, . . . J Maben. 2017. "Exploring the adoption of Schwartz Center Rounds as an organisational innovation to improve staff well-being in England, 2009–2015." *BMJ Open* 7 (1).

Ross, D. 1925. *Aristotle The Nicomachean Ethics: Translated with an Introduction*. Oxford: Oxford University Press.

Rotenstein, LS, MA Ramos, M Torre, JB Segal, MJ Peluso, C Guille, . . . DA Mata. 2016. "Prevalence of depression, depressive symptoms, and suicidal ideation among medical students: A systematic review and meta-analysis." *JAMA* 316 (21):2214–2236.

Rothenberger, D. 2017. "Physician burnout and well-being: A systematic review and framework for action." *Diseases of the Colon & Rectum* 60 (6):567–576.

Shanafelt, T, L Dyrbye, C Sinsky, O Hasan, D Satele, J Sloan, and C West. 2016. "Relationship between clerical burden and characteristics of the electronic environment with physician burnout and professional satisfaction." *Mayo Clinic Proceedings* 9 (7):836–848.

Shanafelt, T, L Dyrbye, and C West. 2017. "Addressing physician burnout: The way forward." *JAMA* 317 (9):901–902.

Smith, B, J Allen-Collinson, C Phoenix, D Brown, and AC Sparkes. 2009. "Dialogue, monologue, and boundary crossing within research encounters: A performative narrative analysis." *International Journal of Sport and Exercise Psychology* 7 (3):342–358.

Topin, J. 2018. "On the other side of physician burnout." *STAT*, 17 May. Accessed 6 August 2019. www.statnews.com/2018/05/17/physician-burnout-working-part-time/.

Welp, A, LL Meier, and T Manser. 2015. "Emotional exhaustion and workload predict clinician-rated and objective patient safety." *Frontiers in Psychology* 5.

West, C, L Dyrbye, P Erwin, and T Shanafelt. 2016. "Interventions to prevent and reduce physician burnout: A systematic review and meta-analysis." *The Lancet* 388 (10057):2272–2281.

West, C, L Dyrbye, and T Shanafelt. 2018. "Physician burnout: Contributors, consequences and solutions (Review)." *Journal of Internal Medicine* 283:516–529.

West, C, A Tan, T Habermann, J Sloan, and T Shanafelt. 2009. "Association of resident fatigue and distress with perceived medical errors." *JAMA* 302:1294–1300.

Wilson, A, C Millard, and I Sabroe. 2019. "Physician narratives of illness." *The Lancet* 394 (10192):20–21.

Wilson, E, A Kenny, and V Dickson-Swift. 2015. "Using blogs as a qualitative health research tool: A scoping review." *International Journal of Qualitative Methods*:1–12.

12 Resilient healthcare in refractory epilepsy

Illuminating successful people-centred patient care

Patti Shih, Janet C Long, Emilie Francis-Auton, Mia Bierbaum, Mona Faris, Robyn Clay-Williams and Frances Rapport

Refractory epilepsy and its treatment: a background

Refractory epilepsy is a complex and chronic condition, where people with seizures are unresponsive to two or more antiepileptic drugs. Resective surgery removes part of the brain cortex triggering the seizures, which can help up to two-thirds of eligible patients achieve seizure freedom (Kwan, Schachter, and Brodie 2011; Jobst and Cascino 2015; Jehi et al. 2015). For many it has led to improved outcomes in patients' employment status, mental health and social integration (Brandalise et al. 2016; Taylor et al. 2011; Spencer et al. 2007; Kanner 2016). Nevertheless, resective surgery remains the most underutilized treatment in refractory epilepsy (Sauro et al. 2015; Engel 2014; Jette, Reid, and Wiebe 2014; Englot 2015).

A situation where a patient with a condition like refractory epilepsy, who would benefit from treatment and yet does not undergo treatment is referred to as the 'treatment gap' (Rapport et al. 2017; Boon et al. 2015). The first treatment gap with this disease applies to the length of time for patients to be correctly diagnosed and referred to a specialist within a Tertiary Epilepsy Centre (TEC). Globally, this is estimated to be around 22 years for patients with refractory epilepsy (Engel 2014; Berg et al. 2003), 17 years specifically, in Australia. The second treatment gap refers to the period of time between a patient's first admission to a TEC and them undergoing surgery. In Australia, this second delay can be anything from six months to two years (Rapport et al. 2017), which is comparable to other international studies (Martínez-Juárez et al. 2017; Hill et al. 2018).

Studies focusing on the treatment gap in refractory epilepsy have primarily aimed to identify treatment barriers, both clinical and in terms of healthcare system and service implementation. For example, the inconsistency in knowledge of surgical treatment among referring general practitioners (GPs) and general neurologists has been found to influence timely referrals (Erba et al. 2012; Cothros, Burneo, and Steven 2016). The delays in pre-surgical evaluations have been cited as including human factors such as a patient's refusal for surgery, resource limitations, and inconsistent workflow in TECs (Anderson et al. 2013; Fois et al. 2016;

Hill et al. 2018). This problematizes the attitude among both patients and health-care professionals (HCPs) towards surgical intervention and has led to suggestions that resective surgery is often a 'last resort' treatment (Berg et al. 2003).

The conventional approach to examine barriers in healthcare, including the challenges of moving patients through the system quickly or involving them in timely surgical discussion, is to undertake a barrier analysis. This kind of analysis examines and identifies direct causes of a problem leading to recommendations to target these causes. The solutions to the conventional treatment barriers in refractory epilepsy tend to be analyzed as top-down, unidirectional approaches to medical interventions, such as recommendations to reinforce early identification and referral through clinical guidelines (Lukmanji et al. 2018; Sauro et al. 2015), or recommendations towards 'streamlining' workflow (Hill et al. 2018). These demonstrate an idealization of a perfect 'end point', where the set goal of surgical uptake can be achieved through a linear progression of activities, with policies and guidelines assumed to be able to predict and constrain human behaviours and decision-making. Moreover, treatment barriers are but one part of the treatment phenomenon, thus a barrier analysis is too narrow in its capacity to address the comprehensive processes and issues facing patients and healthcare professionals in this context.

While the root cause approach tackles obvious barriers to planned procedure, everyday clinical practice is complex. This is illustrated by the difference between 'work-as-imagined' (WAI) and 'work-as-done' (WAD) in the resilient healthcare literature (De Certeau 1984; Braithwaite et al. 2016; Clay-Williams et al. 2015). WAI and WAD is based on the premise that the further a HCP is displaced from direct patient care, the greater the potential for developing a different under-standing about how the work is actually being undertaken. Focusing on health-care policy in epilepsy, and TEC management of the healthcare workforce, HCPs are said to be dealing with WAI, idealizing healthcare functions within planned and systematic processes. However, we know that the treatment of refractory epi-lepsy patients is according to more immediate WAD requirements, where human interaction at the coalface of treatment takes place in an often ad hoc and reac-tive fashion, and where behaviours and responses are often readjusted outside of planned and predicted processes.

In healthcare, we see the ability of HCPs to respond to events and human behav-iours as a strength, an important element of WAD, and their ability to deal with change, contributing clearly to system resilience (Wears, Hollnagel, and Braith-waite 2015; Braithwaite et al. 2017). Resilient thinking highlights the responsive human behaviour at an everyday clinical level that often goes unrecognized, yet ultimately serves the best interests of patients.

In a series of studies examining the implementation of refractory epilepsy treat-ment and care (Rapport et al. 2017; Shih et al. 2018; Mumford et al. 2019; Rap-port et al. 2019; Mitchell et al. 2018), members of the authorship have begun to show the complexity and contextual nature of patient journeys through an often convoluted pathway of healthcare delivery within an ever-changing, adaptive healthcare system (Rapport et al. 2019; Shih et al. 2018).

In this chapter, we seek to clarify what happens during the period of treatment delay, moving the debate of gaps in treatment beyond a simple presentation of barrier or facilitator to smooth patient pathways, and presenting details of a study that examined nuance and complexity in patient experience, alongside the daily clinical workload of HCPs.

Study setting

Our case study of refractory epilepsy treatment took place at two of the three TECs offering resective surgery to refractory epilepsy patients in Sydney, New South Wales (NSW), Australia, between January 2017 and June 2018. The TECs involved were in large metropolitan hospitals, which manage the majority of the diverse and complex (refractory) epilepsy cases referred from across NSW GP and community neurology clinics.

This study utilized qualitative, semi-structured interviews and observations of those at the frontline of patient care, to allow for a comprehensive understanding of WAD in refractory epilepsy treatment. Interviews enabled us to understand HCPs' and patients' perspectives and experiences of work practices, health-care interactions and their interpretations of settings and systems in relation to treatment and care. Observations accompanied interviews and allowed a study researcher (PS) to witness what HCPs and patients do in situ to circumvent or overcome challenges encountered in pursuing resective surgery, quickly and effectively. Together, these methods enabled the study team to access patients' and HCPs' perceptions and experiences of the best possible patient care in the face of refractory epilepsy, and how this might be enabled.

A total of 34 data capture events took place with 18 patients (ten male and eight female, aged 23–64 years) and seven HCPs (four male and three female, ranging in experience from early to senior career professionals and working across the fields of complex epilepsy treatment). Data capture comprised 18 routine clinical observations, 18 patient interviews, and nine HCP interviews.

Study results

Pre-referral challenges and peer support networks

Patients are typically under the care of a GP or general neurologist after their first seizure onset. However, during this period, the identification and referral for refractory epilepsy is often delayed. Our study found a number of barriers for timely referral among our patient cohort, for example, a lack of knowledge about the importance and availability of specialist care, and the lack of proactive referral from treating GPs and community neurologists. The study also revealed that patients received information from personal social networks instead of from typical patient education sources, such as community care or hospital care facilities. Increased knowledge was often facilitated by social support networks through family and friends, patient peer networks, and social media. Patients reported the encouragement of others on the sidelines of care. One patient was finally referred to a TEC after being encouraged by his girlfriend to access a new GP with better knowledge of refractory epilepsy. Another suggested that she was encouraged by a family friend:

> I'd been to this [neurologist] the whole time [since first seizure onset 27 years ago] and [a family friend] said, "I think it might be about time you went and got a second opinion". I was a bit hesitant but I'm glad that I did, because this other younger fellow said to me, "No, I'm not happy with that. You need to go down to [the TEC in] Sydney".
>
> [Patient 12, female, age 49]

Reasons for referral may become more relevant over time, rather than immediately noticeable to treating GPs and community neurologists. For a chronic condition such as epilepsy, response to antiepileptic drugs can be intermittent, thus a specialist referral may only become necessary after a period of time has passed when treating GPs and/or community neurologists become aware that different care may be needed for a certain patient. Furthermore, shifts in the knowledge and attitudes of community HCPs towards treatments such as resective surgery can also affect their referral practices. For example, one patient had been treated under a community neurologist for several decades until things suddenly changed:

> [Neurologist] had mentioned about surgery for epilepsy years ago. About ten, twenty years ago or something. But he said he wasn't sure if they are that good then. Then couple of years ago he said to me that the technology is getting better, the surgeries are getting better and there are better doctors now, so then he got me up here [TEC].
>
> [Patient 20, male, age 53]

The changes in both HCPs' and patients' attitudes and practices towards referral and treatment were facilitated by changes in patients' personal circumstances, the clinicians' confidence in their referral, new knowledge acquired by HCPs or patients about new possibilities for treatment and care, and each patients' level of seizure control. Referrals could be initiated by patients themselves, by HCPs, or by others in the patient's support network. Notably, social networks between patients were also important in revealing available support systems, facilitating access to new information, and helping patients to become proactive in pursuing specialist care.

Online, offline, formal, and informal settings, where patients meet peers with the same or similar medical condition, were useful opportunities for networking. Moreover, referrals, based on the HCP's confidence in the referral process and quality of the technology, were informed by the knowledge of the doctors and the surgery available. In the case of Patient 20 (indicated in the earlier quote), the patient's community neurologist only referred the patient on for surgery when he was confident that the care the patient would receive would be likely to be an improvement on what could be provided in the community setting.

From a WAD perspective, this suggests that we cannot assume that a referral will always lead to a positive patient outcome following surgery. Indeed, when HCPs have reservations about the referral pathway, not referring until these reservations are addressed could be a strong example of 'things going right'.

The facilitation of cultural and attitudinal change

The peer networks of HCPs are crucial to resilient healthcare (McNeil, Brna, and Gordon 2012; Elafros et al. 2013). Knowledge-sharing among clinicians is important for facilitating wider changes in clinical practice. HCPs work in a rapidly changing environment, where the evidence for best practice in epilepsy treatment is constantly being updated. As new drug trials, technological innovation, and treatment approaches emerge to inform research and practice, professional development opportunities become ways of keeping abreast with new knowledge and practices.

An epileptologist in this study (a clinician specializing in epilepsy disease) suggested that there had been a 'paradigm shift' in recent years among HCPs, as the evidence-base for the efficacy of earlier referral for resective surgery had grown. This is partly attributed to the involvement of professional networks in dissemination of information on the topic, through both training and conference opportunities, and links to key sites where new knowledge is shared.

Rather than relying on the shift towards acceptance for earlier referrals, however, some epileptologists said they actively encouraged better referral practices and pathways. Some regularly travelled to regional centres that do not have residential epilepsy and/or neurology specialists, for week-long consultation clinics, or to work with regional colleagues remotely, to increase better referral procedures and information sharing.

> Recently I've been doing telehealth conferencing with [doctors in a regional centre]. There's a neurologist there and if the patients have refractory seizures, we talk about it over the phone, and bring them to [TEC] for further surgical evaluation when it's needed.
>
> [HCP 2, mid-career epileptologist]

This kind of knowledge-spread and uptake by HCPs, as key players in the healthcare system, who provide peer support and actively engage with newly emerging information, is an example of when 'things go right' through human interaction and appropriate engagement with clinical evidence.

Person-centred TEC management

A further period of delay for patients undertaking resective brain surgery after referral to a TEC is the extensive investigation and assessment of surgery eligibility. This time-period poses another challenge (Hill et al. 2018; Martínez-Juárez et al. 2017; Kaiboriboon et al. 2015). The dilemma facing HCPs and patients, as patients spend further, extended periods of time waiting for pre-surgical assessment at the TEC is whether there are more appropriate ways for patients to access surgery and in addition, what support patients and their families will need in the meantime. Delays such as these can prolong poor quality of life and lead to further physical and mental deterioration and to uncertainty and anxiety as patients and HCPs prevaricate about surgical decisions.

The research team undertook a study reviewing issues related to patient quality of life through refractory epilepsy patients' medical records. The review involved 50 patients undergoing surgical evaluation in 2014 and assessed their medical records for a full year, from the same two TECs in NSW involved in this study. The team discovered that patients who underwent surgery spent on average 38.8 weeks between their first TEC assessment and surgical intervention (Mumford et al. 2019). This figure is comparable to studies elsewhere (Martínez-Juárez et al. 2017; Mumford et al. 2019), and the study indicated numerous visits and investigations.

The term 'delay' implies a period of inaction and a stalling of treatment. However, the medical records review study (Mumford et al. 2019) and a further qualitative study of patient experience in the period of time leading up to surgery (Shih et al. 2018) found the pre-surgical period of care in the TEC was intensive and active, involving thorough medical contact and pre-surgical assessment.

The study highlighted that this is a time where patients are verbally prepared for surgery and where tailored treatments occur in the build up to surgery. As shown in our medical records review study, a surgery cohort from the two TECs underwent a drug change on 42% of visits and a dosage change on 37% of visits, clearly impacting patients' quality of life and putting extra strain on their relationships over this time (Mumford et al. 2019). Our previous qualitative results of patient experience in the build up to surgery also suggest that frequent pre-surgical neurological tests put additional strain on patients; however both studies indicate that to a degree this was a necessary element of thorough examination, in order to ensure surgical decision-making would achieve the best result and to ensure lower risk from surgical outcomes (Shih et al. 2018).

Indeed, the pre-surgical period of treatment was seen as vital for HCPs to provide tailored antiepileptic drug management plans and individualized neuropsychological support. HCPs reinforced the need to consider individual circumstances, through patient-centred care approaches, reviews of pre-surgical assessments and seizure-impact on health-related quality of life, before surgery could be offered.

> Patients who may have significant psychiatric comorbidity, or develop mental delay and intellectual impairment, I may try a little harder with medications before going down that route, because of the fact that they may not tolerate the process of being worked up for surgery quite as well, but I still think that everybody needs to be considered. I will generally introduce that concept early, even though we will clearly try ongoing drug trials, because we have so many more medications available to us.
>
> [HCP 3, senior career epileptologist]

The ongoing management of antiepileptic drugs, which takes account person-centred, everyday care needs, enables patients to continue to participate in daily activities. Patients spoke of the benefits of effective drug management tailored to personal circumstances and how their health conditions improved after contact with epileptologists with specialist knowledge.

> [TEC epileptologist would ask] "What kind of job are you in, what's really going to work for you? Because I'm not going to give you a drug that's going to make you drowsy and down if you are in a high stress scenario".
>
> [Patient 11, male, age 39]

Another participant experienced weight-loss from what he felt was a medication side-effect, and he felt he could communicate with HCPs who "listened" and responded as his condition changed.

> [TEC epileptologist] prescribed me one particular medicine and I was not having my meals properly. I strongly believe that it is because of this medication. I lost 10 kilos of my weight. I shared that with doctor, doctor straight away changed my medication. Now I'm gaining weight. The quality of consultation is important. [TEC epileptologist] is very good. She listened to us. What we are thinking, we share with her. She listened to us and straight away and takes a decision. After we touch-base with her, everything goes very smoothly, and I am doing well.
>
> [Patient 7, male, age 40]

Supportive HCP partnerships were fostered by the HCP's willingness to listen and act upon a patient's concerns, which in turn increased the patient's willingness to communicate. While gaining seizure control remains the main treatment goal, HCPs were quick to reinforce that managing a patient's overall quality of life requires a consideration of a variety of psychosocial factors beyond seizure control, and how to communicate these issues to patients. Several patients valued the engagement with neuropsychological and counselling support services provided by TECs, before and after surgery.

While a cautionary approach to treatment contributed to what may seem a 'delay' to timely uptake of surgery, therefore, the key priority for HCPs and patients was person-centred care and the need to ensure the odds of surgical success were high, while minimizing the chance of complications post-surgery, such as cognitive deficits. This was seen by all participants as good practice and considered the most appropriate approach, as opposed to a singular focus to clinical outcome-delivery.

Discussion

Existing literature considers referral delays in refractory epilepsy to be a one-dimensional, negative phenomenon, where patients are simply not getting the right treatment in time, or in high enough numbers. But simply targeting treatment barriers, using a barrier analysis, only enables understanding of one part of the complex phenomenon. Using qualitative research, this study eluci-dated the 'real world' scenarios of everyday clinical practice using a refractory epilepsy case study, and contrasted people's views of WAI with WAD, as a result. Rather than focusing on expectations of what 'should' happen in an idealized way, the study focused on what 'is' happening, and as a consequence, the value of both barriers and facilitators to quicker patient mobility through the system. As a result, the study team considered both positive and negative aspects of treatment processes and patient pathways, as part of the phenom-enon: 'delays in treatment'. This has enabled an understanding of how success-ful treatment trajectories are facilitated around and beyond root cause failures, over time.

As the study suggests, it has often been assumed that patients would and should know about treatment options, and that HCPs should be aware of and accept the most up-to-date research evidence, acting efficiently and effectively. Rather, as central actors within the healthcare system, patients and families have had to be self-informed about treatment, while HCPs have had to try a range of new ways to self-educate and disseminate new research within their professional networks. HCPs in the community are also clearly trying to manage patients in their care, which appears to extend the time that patients remain under GP or community neurologists, before being referred on to a TEC.

While the assertion that a speedy assessment for resective surgery is ideal (WAI), in reality it is more complex than that. The willingness to be flexible and more considered in terms of treatment progress is often more effective in this context (WAD). Successful treatment includes thorough investigations of each patient's condition to ensure that risks and deficits are minimized, and that the most accurate medical information informs treatment decision-making, rather than proceeding to surgery with less odds of success and greater risk of complica-tions (Shih et al. 2018). Instead of a prescriptive approach to the singular pursuit of timely surgical uptake, which risks more complications, the focus, in reality, is on wider aspects of psychosocial health and patient wellbeing. It is also a multidi-mensional approach that recognizes the interdependence between factors such as the health of the whole person, not only their ability to achieve seizure freedom. While resource challenges, transitions through care and waiting times are often partly to blame for longer delays, investigations need to be thorough and person-centred; this holistic approach to care is crucial.

The resilient properties of the healthcare system outlined in this chapter, as exemplified in WAD in this context, are embedded within the ability of people and treatment practices to adapt in response to change. At the same time people need to be drivers of change, rather than simply adhering to an idealized clinical process. These insights can help us understand 'what goes right' and as a result, how we may need to radically rethink the current approaches to dealing with treatment gaps in refractory epilepsy, rather than concentrating on 'what goes wrong'.

References

Anderson, C, E Noble, R Mani, K Lawler, and J Pollard. 2013. "Epilepsy surgery: Factors that affect patient decision-making in choosing or deferring a procedure." *Epilepsy Research and Treatment* 2013:13. doi: 10.1155/2013/309284.

Berg, A, J Langfitt, S Shinnar, B Vickrey, M Sperling, T Walczak, C Bazil, S Pacia, and S Spencer. 2003. "How long does it take for partial epilepsy to become intractable?" *Neurology* 60 (2):186–190.

Boon, P, P Ryvlin, J Wheless, and K Kawai. 2015. "Treating drug-resistant epilepsy – Why are we waiting?" *European Neurological Review* 10 (2):171–175.

Braithwaite, J, K Churruca, LA Ellis, J Long, R Clay-Williams, N Damen, J Herkes, C Pomare, and K Ludlow. 2017. *Complexity Science in Healthcare – Aspirations, Approaches, Applications and Accomplishments: A White Paper*. Sydney, Australia: Australian Institute of Health Innovation, Macquarie University.

Braithwaite, J, R Clay-Williams, G Hunt, and R Wears. 2016. "Understanding resilient clinical practices in emergency department ecosystems." In *Resilient Health Care*, edited by J Braithwaite, R Wears, and E Hollnagel. Farnham: Ashgate Publishing, Ltd.

Brandalise, M, G Barbosa, R Centeno, E Yacubian, and G de Araujo Filho. 2016. "Depressive and anxiety symptoms exert negative impact on resilience to stressful events in patients with refractory temporal lobe epilepsy with late seizure recurrence after surgery." *Journal of Psychology & Psychotherapy* 6 (269):2161–2487.

Clay-Williams, R, J Johnson, D Debono, and J Braithwaite. 2015. "The path from policy to practice: Resilience of everyday work in acute settings." In *Managing Change: From Health Policy to Practice*, edited by S Waldorff, A Pedersen, E Ferlie, and L Fitzgerald. London: Palgrave Macmillan.

Cothros, N, J Burneo, and D Steven. 2016. "Knowledge and attitudes about epilepsy surgery among family doctors in Ontario." *Canadian Journal of Neurological Sciences* 43 (5):672–677.

De Certeau, M. 1984. *The Practice of Everyday Life*. Berkeley: University of California Press.

Elafros, M, J Mulenga, E Mbewe, A Haworth, E Chomba, M Atadzhanov, and G Birbeck. 2013. "Peer support groups as an intervention to decrease epilepsy-associated stigma." *Epilepsy & Behavior* 27 (1):188–192.

Engel, J. 2014. "Approaches to refractory epilepsy." *Annals of Indian Academy of Neurology* 17 (S1):S12.

Englot, D. 2015. "The persistent under-utilization of epilepsy surgery." *Epilepsy Research* 118:68–69.

Erba, G, L Moja, E Beghi, P Messina, and E Pupillo. 2012. "Barriers toward epilepsy surgery: A survey among practicing neurologists." *Epilepsia* 53 (1):35–43.

Fois, C, S Kovac, A Khalil, G Uzuner, B Diehl, T Wehner, J Duncan, and M Walker. 2016. "Predictors for being offered epilepsy surgery: 5-year experience of a tertiary referral centre." *Journal of Neurology, Neurosurgery, and Psychiatry* 87 (2):209–211.

Hill, C, J Raab, D Roberts, T Lucas, J Pollard, A Kheder, B Litt, and K Davis. 2018. "Addressing barriers to surgical evaluation for patients with epilepsy." *Epilepsy & Behavior* 86:1–5.

Jehi, L, D Friedman, C Carlson, G Cascino, S Dewar, C Elger, J Engel Jr, R Knowlton, R Kuzniecky, A McIntosh, T O'Brien, D Spencer, M Sperling, G Worrell, B Bingaman, J Gonzalez-Martinez, W Doyle, and J French. 2015. "The evolution of epilepsy surgery between 1991 and 2011 in nine major epilepsy centers across the United States, Germany, and Australia." *Epilepsia* 56 (10):1526–1533.

Jette, N, A Reid, and S Wiebe. 2014. "Surgical management of epilepsy." *Canadian Medical Association Journal* 186 (13):997–1004.

Jobst, B, and G Cascino. 2015. "Resective epilepsy surgery for drug-resistant focal epilepsy: A review." *JAMA* 313 (3):285–293.

Kaiboriboon, K, A Malkhachroum, A Zrik, A Daif, N Schiltz, D Labiner, and S Lhatoo. 2015. "Epilepsy surgery in the United States: Analysis of data from the national association of epilepsy centers." *Epilepsy Research* 116:105–109. doi: 10.1016/j.eplepsyres.2015.07.007.

Kanner, A. 2016. "Management of psychiatric and neurological comorbidities in epilepsy." *Nature Reviews Neurology* 12 (2):106.

Kwan, P, S Schachter, and M Brodie. 2011. "Drug-resistant epilepsy." *New England Journal of Medicine* 365 (10):919–926.

Lukmanji, S, K Altura, B Rydenhag, K Malmgren, S Wiebe, and N Jetté. 2018. "Accuracy of an online tool to assess appropriateness for an epilepsy surgery evaluation – A population-based Swedish study." *Epilepsy Research* 145:140–144.

Martínez-Juárez, IE, B Funes, JC Moreno-Castellanos, E Bribiesca-Contreras, V Martínez-Bustos, L Zertuche-Ortuño, LE Hernández-Vanegas, LH Ronquillo, S Rizvi, and W Adam. 2017. "A comparison of waiting times for assessment and epilepsy surgery between a Canadian and a Mexican referral center." *Epilepsia Open* 2 (4):453–458.

McNeil, K, P Brna, and K Gordon. 2012. "Epilepsy in the Twitter era: A need to re-tweet the way we think about seizures." *Epilepsy & Behavior* 23 (3):127–130.

Mitchell, R, G Herkes, A Nikpour, A Bleasel, P Shih, S Vagholkar, and F Rapport. 2018. "Examining health service utilization, hospital treatment cost, and mortality of individuals with epilepsy and status epilepticus in New South Wales, Australia 2012–2016." *Epilepsy & Behavior* 79:9–16.

Mumford, V, F Rapport, P Shih, R Mitchell, A Bleasel, A Nikpour, G Herkes, A MacRae, M Bartley, S Vagholkar, and J Braithwaite. 2019. "Promoting faster pathways to surgery: A clinical audit of patients with refractory epilepsy." *BMC Neurology* 19 (1):29.

Rapport, F, P Shih, M Faris, A Nikpour, G Herkes, A Bleasel, M Kerr, R Clay-Williams, V Mumford, and J Braithwaite. 2019. "Determinants of health and wellbeing in refractory epilepsy and surgery: The Patient Reported, ImpleMentation sciEnce (PRIME) model." *Epilepsy & Behavior* 92:79–89.

Rapport, F, P Shih, R Mitchell, A Nikpour, A Bleasel, G Herkes, S Vagholkar, and V Mumford. 2017. "Better evidence for earlier assessment and surgical intervention for refractory epilepsy (The BEST study): A mixed methods study protocol." *BMJ Open* 7 (8).

Sauro, KM, S Wiebe, E Perucca, J French, C Dunkley, A de Marinis, M Kirkpatrick, and N Jette. 2015. "Developing clinical practice guidelines for epilepsy: A report from the ILAE Epilepsy Guidelines Working Group." *Epilepsia*. doi: 10.1111/epi.13217.

Shih, P, A Nikpour, A Bleasel, G Herkes, R Mitchell, R Seah, V Mumford, J Braithwaite, S Vagholkar, and F Rapport. 2018. "Leading up to saying 'yes': A qualitative study of refractory epilepsy patients' experiences of pre-surgical investigation." *Epilepsy & Behavior* 83:36–43.

Spencer, SS, AT Berg, BG Vickrey, MR Sperling, CW Bazil, S Haut, JT Langfitt, TS Walczak, and O Devinsky. 2007. "Health-related quality of life over time since resective epilepsy surgery." *Annals of Neurology* 62 (4):327–334.

Taylor, RS, JW Sander, RJ Taylor, and GA Baker. 2011. "Predictors of health-related quality of life and costs in adults with epilepsy: A systematic review." *Epilepsia* 52 (12):2168–2180.

Wears, R, E Hollnagel, and J Braithwaite. 2015. *Resilient Health Care: The Resilience of Everyday Clinical Work*. Vol. 2. Farnham: Ashgate Publishing, Ltd.

Part 3

Solutions

This is the point where we enter the final section of the book, Part 3, Solutions. Here, we move from 'ideas about health and personhood' in Part 1, and 'notions for change' in Part 2, to 'positive change'. Part 3 examines: new frameworks for change management and the management of uncertainty based on complexity science (Lanham et al.); simulation, debriefing, and reflection for healthcare teams and their improvement (Patterson and Deutsch); building resilience through cross-boundary teaming (Nakamura et al.); positive identity construction and the active role of the 'sensemaker' (Churruca et al.); the value of implementation science for routinising genomics in practice (Best et al.); and Soft Systems Methodology by which to evaluate and enact healthcare change (Augustsson et al.).

Part 3 brings together a triangulation of ideas – a combination of the extensive knowledge put forward in this book. In taking forward views around 'positive change', we can discern ways that can transform not only the systems in which healthcare professionals work and patients are treated, but also the methodologies and methods that underpin those systems and services. Part 3 chapters describe methods that can be applied to understand, evaluate, and translate research findings into practical implementable solutions to real world healthcare problems. Indeed, Part 3 introduces the reader to an array of exciting new qualitative tools and features, such as: qualitative models for system improvement (Augustsson et al.); surveys and process maps that enable 'deep-dive' assessments of clinical activities and outcomes (Best et al.); and new analytical frameworks to clarify, understand, and work with complex systems and services (Churruca et al., Lanham et al. and Patterson and Deutsch).

This all paves the way in turn for a final chapter, Chapter 19, Conclusion. There, we will bring the whole volume's perspectives – the authors' and editors' collective writings on transforming healthcare through qualitative research – into focus.

13 Sensemaking as a strategy for managing uncertainty

Change and surprise in hospital settings

Holly J Lanham, Jacqueline A Pugh, David C Aron and Luci K Leykum

A hospital is a fluid world characterized by uncertainty, change, and surprise. These difficult-to-manage features result from the nonlinear interdependencies that exist among component parts of a complex adaptive system (Driebe and McDaniel Jr 2005). As Weick stated in his seminal work on the Mann Gulch Disaster,

> In a fluid world, wise people know that they don't fully understand what is happening right now, because they have never seen precisely this event before. Extreme confidence and extreme caution both can destroy what organizations most need in changing times, namely, curiosity, openness, and complex sensing. . . . It is this sense in which wisdom, which avoids extremes, improves adaptability.
>
> (Weick 1993, 641)

We have studied healthcare settings as complex adaptive systems for decades. We use this work to frame our understanding of complex adaptive systems, and how to approach improving these systems, using the creation of collaborative interprofessional patient-partnered care teams as an example.

Hospitals are complex adaptive systems characterized not only by nonlinearity, but also by diverse individuals who interact and learn (Jordan et al. 2009). An example of diverse individuals in a hospital includes the different members of the hospital care team caring for a patient: physicians, nurses, respiratory therapists, physical therapists, social workers, pharmacists, and other health professions, who all bring different backgrounds, experiences, and professional values to the team. As this group interacts in caring for patients, they exchange and process information, learn, and adapt their behaviour over time. As individuals interact, dynamically stable patterns of organizing develop over time (Kauffman 1996). This self-organization can be seen, for example, after a new inpatient physician team is formed at an academic medical centre. The individuals may have been assigned, but the interactions among the members have not been established except in the most general way. The attending (lead) physician, resident, intern, and medical students quickly learn their roles and role-based expectations through interactions as a newly formed team.

Additionally, complex adaptive systems are characterized by emergence. Emergence has many definitions (Barabási and Albert 1999; Goldstein 2011; Holland 1992; Lichtenstein and Plowman 2009; Miller and Page 2009), but the common thread among these definitions is that emergence is a process through which patterns of system behaviour or global-level structures arise from local-level component interactions. The concept of emergence gives us a way to think about system level properties that cannot be understood by examining the components of the system individually. The nonlinearities and emergent dynamics in complex adaptive systems lead to uncertainty and surprise.

Our work demonstrates the importance of relationships (Finley et al. 2013; Lanham et al. 2009; McAllister et al. 2014) and the role of sensemaking in managing uncertainty, change, and surprise in healthcare delivery systems (Jordan et al. 2009; Lanham et al. 2013; Leykum et al. 2015; Leykum, Lanham, Provost et al. 2014; Leykum et al. 2012). For instance, one of our studies found trust and reflection time to be associated with sensemaking as assessed by practice member surveys administered in 36 United States (US) primary care practices (Lanham et al. 2016). Another one of our studies found that patients who were cared for by inpatient care teams with effective relationships and sensemaking had shorter stays and fewer complications than patients who were cared for by teams with less effective relationships and sensemaking (Leykum et al. 2015; McAllister et al. 2014). It is through social interactions and relationships that people are able to make sense of uncertainty, take effective action (Weick 1993, 1995), and improvise if needed (McKenna, Leykum, and McDaniel Jr 2013). To improve the performance of clinical systems, we must improve patients' and providers' ability to interact with each other in the face of uncertainty.

The application of complexity science helps us recognize the inherent uncertainty in hospital systems. It also brings to focus the role of interdependencies in healthcare systems in managing uncertainty (Afifi and Afifi 2015; Boisot and Child 1999; Leykum, Lanham, Pugh et al. 2014; McDaniel Jr 2007). While these interdependencies include the processes of care and resources available, they also include the social structure, communication behaviours, and relationships between patients and providers (Leykum, Lanham, Pugh et al. 2014). Figure 13.1 illustrates our view of how these constructs are connected. Communication and relationships are crucial to managing uncertainty because they provide the foundation for interactions that lead to effective shared mental models and actions based on those shared mental models (Leykum, Lanham, Pugh et al. 2014; McDaniel Jr 2007). Asking questions of their provider team is one way that patients make sense of their clinical situation. Diagnosing a patient is sensemaking in that it is a social process through which providers assimilate information, assign meaning to external cues, and arrive at a shared understanding of a patient's clinical situation. However, sensemaking is larger than asking a question or making a diagnosis, particularly in inpatient ward rounds, as it includes considering the overall trajectory

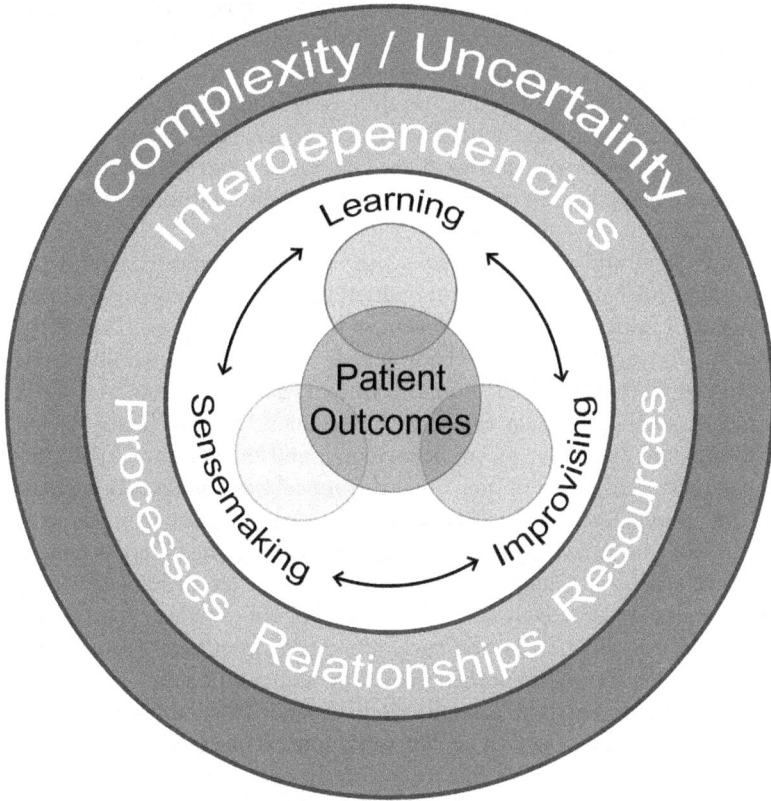

Figure 13.1 Managing complexity and uncertainty in healthcare delivery systems.

Source: Authors' own work.

of a whole-person's illness (as opposed to the biomedical disease) over a relatively short period of time.

Complex adaptive systems make demands on those who deal with them. We know intuitively and have confirmed from research that change and surprise are fundamental aspects of the world in which we live. Instead of conceptualizing social systems as mechanistic with predictable dynamics that need to be discovered then controlled, we now understand that they are self-organizing systems with properties, both predictable and unpredictable, that emerge from the nonlinear interactions of individuals (Miller and Page 2009). This means that attentiveness to the interactions and relationships among the parts of a complex system is critical to understanding and improving its structure and function (Newman, Barabási, and Watts 2006). Thus, improving the individual parts of a complex system will not be as effective as efforts that include improving how the parts of a complex system relate with and impact on each other. It also means that transformational improvement of our healthcare system may require us to abandon our traditional linear based tools of healthcare delivery, open up the system to the patients it serves, and apply standards of excellence in healthcare delivery (Berwick 2010). Similarly, we must also shift away from the mindset of healthcare as a product and toward one of healthcare as a service, and develop improvement approaches that acknowledge this shift. This raises interesting questions about the contrasting approaches of standardization and customization (Mannion and Exworthy 2017).

We must have the ability to make sense of complex inputs (large in number and interdependent) and extract information from data and create meaning from information. Multiple theoretical constructs have been developed and applied to understand the set of issues around how people deal with change and surprise. We acknowledge the work scholars from diverse academic disciplines are conducting around this same and similar complex phenomenon trying to better understand how to improve cognitive, social, behavioural, and organizational performance. How is sensemaking different from other theoretical frameworks seeking to understand how people manage change and surprise? Are we guilty of fitting facts to a frame, as Klein et al. (2007) describe in their critique on the different frames used to examine this issue? Call it what you will, but there are certain skills and attitudes one needs to effectively deal with uncertainty in complex adaptive systems.

Relational coordination is one such framework from the organizational literature. Relational coordination consists of relating and communicating for the purpose of task integration (Gittell, Godfrey, and Thistlethwaite 2013). This framework has been applied in similar work contexts as sensemaking; however, the main focus of relational coordination is on the effective coordination and integration of interdependent work tasks. High reliability is another framework from the organizational literature that is applied in similar contexts. High reliability organizations are organizations that operate in complex, high-hazard domains for long periods of time without serious accidents or catastrophic failures (Christianson et al. 2011; Weick, Sutcliffe, and Obstfeld 2008). These organizations focus on standardization and failure prevention, whereas a sensemaking lens assumes failures to be unavoidable unexpected events and, thus, emphasizes the contextual conditions required for interpersonal interactions that will lead to safe and effective future actions. Finally, a naturalistic decision-making lens has been applied to the study of how people make decisions and perform cognitively complex functions in demanding, real world situations (Klein 2008; Zsambok and Klein 2014). This framework emerged at the intersection of human factors engineering and decision researchers in organizations and is focused on how people make tough decisions under difficult circumstances. Each of these frameworks (and there are many others we do not mention) add to the overall conversation on managing change in complex environments, and they share an acknowledgement of the importance of social interactions in system function. Our choice to use a sensemaking lens derives from our assumptions about the nature of hospitals as complex adaptive systems and the tools and strategies suited for such systems.

Sensemaking

The complexity of the challenges faced in healthcare requires a new paradigm for understanding and addressing them. Our group has approached this problem from a complex systems perspective, considering specifically the relationship systems among the people in healthcare settings and the contexts for sensemaking, or how people assign meaning to experiences. As Weick remind us, "sensemaking is a diagnostic process directed at constructing plausible interpretations of ambiguous cues that are sufficient to sustain action" (Weick 2005, 57). A recent study of between-hospital differences in surgical mortality found that a major contributor to patient death was how quickly complications were recognized and addressed (Ghaferi, Birkmeyer, and Dimick 2009). Another study attributed the inability to see and improve interdependence at a pediatric cardiac surgery centre as a major aspect of failed sensemaking, resulting in preventable deaths (Weick and Sutcliffe 2003). Our own studies contribute additional knowledge about specific relationship characteristics that are needed in healthcare delivery settings (Finley et al. 2013; Lanham et al. 2009; McAllister et al. 2014). Positive relationships among team members provide a foundation for effective collaboration characterized by high psychological safety, a shared belief that the team is safe for interpersonal risk taking, and the capacity to develop and adapt shared mental models (Edmondson 1999).

Building a system of care that positively influences how patients, families, and providers make sense of their world is critical for improving hospital care. Sensemaking and its association with inpatient outcomes demonstrates its importance to the delivery of safe and efficient hospital care (Leykum et al. 2015). Through sensemaking, patients and providers co-create meaning from their experiences and come to a shared understanding of what is happening and why. This shared understanding becomes the platform for effective care decisions and actions. Relationships that are marked by trust, respect, mindfulness, and heedfulness foster the development of a shared understanding (Lanham et al. 2016; Leykum et al. 2015; Lanham et al. 2009; McAllister et al. 2014). This insight is critical for improving complex adaptive systems, for two key reasons. First, change efforts must take into account how individuals relate to each other and make sense of what is happening as part of interventions to improve system function. Second, improvement efforts themselves introduce change and uncertainty. Sensemaking around the improvement intervention as it is implemented is necessary for effective update and adaptation.

Collaborative interprofessional patient-partnered care

We provide an example of a relationship and sensemaking-focused care delivery model grounded in complex adaptive systems thinking. Collaborative interprofessional patient-partnered care is a patient-partnered care model that engages interprofessional teams and hospitalized patients and families to co-create care plans. It is grounded in a complex adaptive system-understanding of healthcare delivery, building on patient-partnered, interprofessional approaches by making explicit the importance of relationships and sensemaking in the delivery of effective care. With this approach, patients, families, and providers partner in creating high-quality care, integrated across disciplines and responsive to individual patients' needs (Batalden et al. 2016). Rather than developing plans in silos, diverse health professionals come to the bedside. Ward rounds are transformed into discussions with patients and families about goals of care, which in turn drive diagnostic and therapeutic plans. These discussions lead to more effective sensemaking, and to improved care. Patients receive the most appropriate care because their preferences, goals, and health issues and concerns are known by the entire team. Care transitions improve because needs are better understood. Shared understanding enables errors or clinical changes to be quickly recognized, leading to fewer errors and complications, and better outcomes.

The collaborative interprofessional patient-partnered care model contains several key components that foster the co-creation of the shared care plan. These components can be discussed in terms of changes to the interdependencies within healthcare systems, such as the *processes*, *resources*, and *relationships*.

- **Patient involvement in the care plan** – In collaborative interprofessional, patient-partnered care, patients are active partners in the development of the care plan. This happens primarily during ward rounds, which are transformed from the traditional hallway or bedside rounds where providers talk about the patient, to a conversation where various options are discussed with the patient. This change to the usual ward round process emphasizes the importance of relationships among the members of the care team but also between the care team and patients and their families. The interprofessional component is critical and may range from the entire team of providers going 'around the circle' to discuss aspects of care, to smaller subgroups on days when pharmacy, physical therapy, or care coordination is not present. Decisions are made at the bedside rather than at a nursing station or physician workroom, with a clear, shared understanding of not only *what* the plan is, but *why* it is being pursued. The resource burden of convening all members of the team for daily bedside ward rounds can be substantial when compared to usual care. However, once established, the benefits to patient care and team performance are usually recognized quickly.
- **Communication of care goals** – Large, poster-sized 'Post-it notes' or white boards placed in patients' rooms are used to communicate goals of care, relevant diagnoses, and each day's care plan to everyone. Each day, resolved issues or completed tests are crossed off the board, and new items are added, allowing patients, families, and providers to look back at the care plan evolution. This process change requires minimal resources and places emphasis on clear communication of patient care goals.
- **Team reflection sessions** – Daily reflective sessions allow the team to reflect on their performance as a team, discussing what is going well and what can be improved in terms of their communication and interactions with patients

and each other. If needed, they can discuss patient-specific follow-up items. This change in process requires resources in terms of care team member time. However, the return on this investment can be profound in terms of team member interactions and relationships. Not only does time to reflect on team performance shape the relationships among team members, but it also builds psychological safety in teams, an important attribute of teams that effectively make sense of change, surprise, and uncertainty (Edmondson 2003).

- **Safety checklist** – We utilize a safety checklist reviewed daily during interprofessional bedside ward rounds. This checklist contains items that are relevant to all hospitalized patients (e.g., mobility, access, catheters, prophylaxis for deep-vein thrombosis) and items that are specific to each patient. At the end of the checklist are two items called 'concerns' and 'contingencies'. These two items are taken from our research on sensemaking in inpatient care settings. They allow the team first to identify and share any potential issues, and then develop contingency plans for events that might occur that day. Patients and families also know what events or symptoms they should be aware of. The discussion of concerns and contingencies has been associated with fewer in-hospital complications (Leykum et al. 2015). This process change focuses on patient safety through improving sensemaking about each hospitalized patient. It brings together the care team to engage specifically around concerns and contingencies, facilitating improved relationships among care team members as a positive side effect.
- **Geographic localization** – Each team's patients are co-located in specific geographical areas. Geographic localization may not be feasible from a process or resource perspective in all contexts, or all of the time in specific contexts. However, even partial co-localization facilitates a consistent interprofessional team caring for a group of patients, enabling relationships to develop and improve among care team members and between care team members and patients.

The process map in Figure 13.2 demonstrates how collaborative interprofessional patient-partnered care fosters improved patient outcomes through changes in processes, resources, and relationships focused on improving sensemaking about hospitalized patients.

Collaborative Interprofessional patient-partnered care and usual care contrasted

Table 13.1 summarizes the key differences between usual and collaborative interprofessional patient-partnered care in inpatient care settings.

The diagrams in Figure 13.3 highlight the communication flows with usual (left) and collaborative interprofessional patient-partnered (right) care models, illustrating how interactions and information-flow in the collaborative model enable the co-creation of patient-centred, shared care plans.

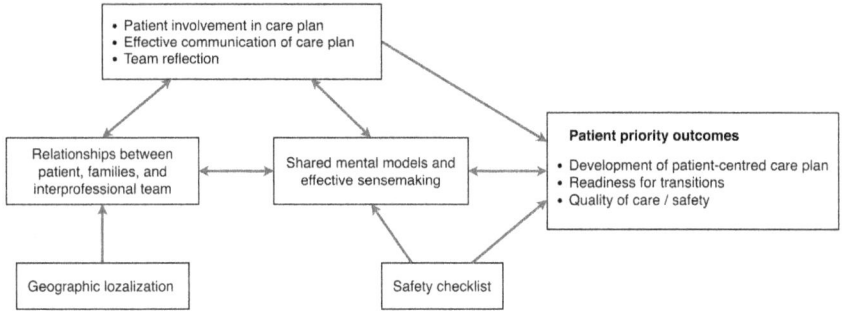

Figure 13.2 Process map of collaborative interprofessional patient-partnered care.
Source: Authors' own work.

Table 13.1 Differences between usual and collaborative care

	Usual care	Collaborative care
Patients	May or may not be active part of planning.	Patients as partners in developing the care plan.
Goals of care	Set by physicians, may not be clear to patients.	Jointly developed, transparent, communicated.
Workflow	Within silos.	Explicitly coordinated between professions.
Communication	Ad hoc, inconsistent.	Part of expected workflow, interprofessional communication embedded in daily schedules.
Philosophy	Centred around individual provider needs, process-based.	Patient-partnered, emphasis on the team.

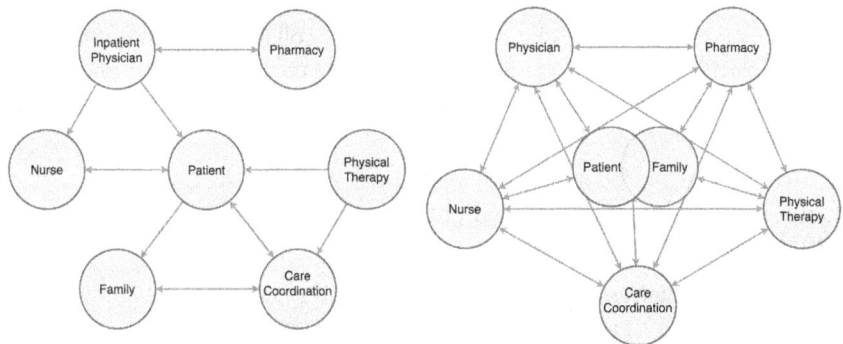

Figure 13.3 Communication flows with usual (left) and collaborative interprofessional patient-partnered (right) care models.
Source: Authors' own work.

What collaborative interprofessional patient-partnered care has shown

Our data from studies of inpatient teams suggest that the benefit from collaborative care implementation is substantial. Providers were initially concerned that these ward rounds would be more time consuming. However, based on our observations of ward rounds on collaborative and 'usual care' teams, we found no difference in the amount of time spent per patient during ward rounds between the collaborative and usual care models, with all teams spending approximately 17 minutes and 15 seconds per patient. However, who spoke during ward rounds differed greatly between team types. Physicians (including residents and medical students) on usual care teams spoke 93% of the time. Patients spoke only 5% of time, and other health professionals contributed only 2% of the time. In contrast, on collaborative interprofessional patient-partnered care teams, physicians spoke only 54% of the time. Patients and family spoke 17% of the time, with 29% of the time contributed by other healthcare professions.

We also compared the Hospital Consumer Assessment of Healthcare Providers and Systems (HCAHPS) survey scores (Centre for Medicare & Medicaid Services 2017) assessing patient experience between the collaborative and usual care teams over a one-year period. HCAHPS is a standardized, publicly reported survey that is used nationally by hospitals in the United States, consisting of 27 questions that ask patients to rate aspects of their hospital stay (Centre for Medicare & Medicaid Services 2017). Scores of patients cared for on collaborative teams were significantly higher than usual care teams. The largest gains were seen on the following items: staff described medication side effects (54.3% versus 66.7% strongly agreed); staff took preferences into account (42.2% versus 49.6% strongly agreed); nurses explained things understandably (76.1% versus 84.2% strongly agreed); treated with courtesy and respect by doctors (86.3% versus 91.7% strongly agreed). The only item which patients who were cared for on a collaborative care team rated lower, was whether pain was well-controlled during their hospitalization (62.9% versus 55.8%). One interpretation of this result is that collaborative care teams were perhaps talking with patients more about their pain levels and were then less likely to administer medications.

Summary

We have used our work in healthcare systems to demonstrate the role of sense-making in improving complex adaptive systems. Complex adaptive systems are inherently uncertain (Greenhalgh and Papoutsi 2018). Efforts to change these systems increase uncertainty by changing how work is organized, and outcomes of these efforts are not predictably clear. Because of this inherent unpredictability, developing capacity for people to make effective sense of what is happening is critical for good outcomes. Relationships, social interactions, and communication are the foundation for effective sensemaking. Enabling effective sensemaking is an important aspect of managing change. Strategies to improve relationships, provide time and space for conversation, and use of tools to promote communication all contribute to effective sensemaking. In turn, sensemaking improves our ability to change the way we deliver care.

References

Afifi, T, and W Afifi. 2015. *Uncertainty, Information Management, and Disclosure Decisions: Theories and Applications*. New York: Routledge.

Barabási, A-L, and R Albert. 1999. "Emergence of scaling in random networks." *Science* 286 (5439):509–512. doi: 10.1126/science.286.5439.509.

Batalden, M, P Batalden, P Margolis, M Seid, G Armstrong, L Opipari-Arrigan, and H Hartung. 2016. "Coproduction of healthcare service." *BMJ Quality & Safety* 25 (7):509–517.

Berwick, DM. 2010. *Escape Fire: Designs for the Future of Health Care*. San Francisco: John Wiley & Sons, Ltd.

Boisot, M, and J Child. 1999. "Organizations as Adaptive Systems in Complex Environments: The Case of China." *Organization Science* 10 (3):237–252.

Centre for Medicare & Medicaid Services. 2017. "HCAHPS: Patients' Perspectives of Care Survey." Last Modified 21 December 2017. Accessed August 2019. www.cms.gov/Medicare/Quality-Initiatives-Patient-Assessment-Instruments/HospitalQualityInits/Hospital-HCAHPS.html.

Christianson, MK, KM Sutcliffe, MA Miller, and TJ Iwashyna. 2011. "Becoming a high reliability organization." *Critical Care* 15 (6):314.

Driebe, DJ, and RR McDaniel Jr. 2005. "Complexity, uncertainty and surprise: An integrated view." In *Uncertainty and Surprise in Complex Systems*, edited by DJ Driebe and RR McDaniel. Berlin: Springer. 19–30.

Edmondson, AC. 1999. "Psychological safety and learning behavior in work teams." *Administrative Science Quarterly* 44 (2):350–383.

Edmondson, AC. 2003. "Speaking up in the operating room: How team leaders promote learning in interdisciplinary action teams." *Journal of Management Studies* 40 (6):1419–1452.

Finley, EP, JA Pugh, HJ Lanham, LK Leykum, J Cornell, P Veerapaneni, and M Parchman. 2013. "Relationship quality and patient-assessed quality of care in VA primary care clinics: Development and validation of the work relationships scale." *The Annals of Family Medicine* 11 (6):543–549.

Ghaferi, AA, JD Birkmeyer, and JB Dimick. 2009. "Complications, failure to rescue, and mortality with major inpatient surgery in medicare patients." *Annals of Surgery* 250 (6):1029–1034.

Gittell, JH, M Godfrey, and J Thistlethwaite. 2013. "Interprofessional collaborative practice and relational coordination: Improving healthcare through relationships." *Journal of Interprofessional Care* 27 (3):210–213. doi: 10.3109/13561820.2012.730564.

Goldstein, J. 2011. "Emergence in complex systems." In *The Sage Handbook of Complexity and Management*, edited by P Allen, S Maguire and B McKelvey. London: Sage.

Greenhalgh, T, and C Papoutsi. 2018. "Studying complexity in health services research: Desperately seeking an overdue paradigm shift." *BMC Medicine* 16 (95). doi: 10.1186/s12916-018-1089-4.

Holland, JH. 1992. "Complex adaptive systems." *Daedalus* 121 (1):17–30.

Jordan, ME, HJ Lanham, B Crabtree, PA Nutting, WL Miller, KC Stange, and RR McDaniel Jr. 2009. "The role of conversation in health care interventions: Enabling sensemaking and learning." *Implementation Science* 4 (15). doi: 10.1186/1748-5908-4-15.

Kauffman, SA. 1996. *At Home in the Universe: The Search for the Laws of Self-Organization and Complexity*. New York: Oxford University Press.

Klein, G. 2008. "Naturalistic decision making." *Human Factors* 50 (3):456–460.

Klein, G, JK Phillips, EL Rall, and DA Peluso. 2007. "A data – frame theory of sense-making." In *Expertise Out of Context: Proceedings of the Sixth International Conference on Naturalistic Decision Making*, edited by RR Hoffman. New York: Lawrence Erlbaum Associates. 113–155.

Lanham, HJ, LK Leykum, BS Taylor, CJ McCannon, C Lindberg, and RT Lester. 2013. "How complexity science can inform scale-up and spread in health care: Understanding the role of self-organization in variation across local contexts." *Social Science & Medicine* 93:194–202.

Lanham, HJ, RR McDaniel Jr, BF Crabtree, WL Miller, KC Stange, AF Tallia, and PA Nutting. 2009. "How improving practice relationships among clinicians and nonclinicians can improve quality in primary care." *The Joint Commission Journal on Quality and Patient Safety* 35 (9):457–466.

Lanham, HJ, RF Palmer, LK Leykum, RR McDaniel Jr, PA Nutting, KC Stange, . . . CR Jaén. 2016. "Trust and reflection in primary care practice redesign." *Health Services Research* 51 (4):1489–1514.

Leykum, LK, H Chesser, HJ Lanham, P Carla, R Palmer, T Ratcliffe, . . . JA Pugh. 2015. "The association between sensemaking during physician team rounds and hospitalized patients' outcomes." *Journal of General Internal Medicine* 30 (12):1821–1827. doi: 10.1007/s11606-015-3377-4.

Leykum, LK, P Kumar, M Parchman, RR McDaniel Jr, HJ Lanham, and M Agar. 2012. "Use of an agent-based model to understand clinical systems." *Journal of Artificial Societies and Social Simulation* 15 (3):2.

Leykum, LK, HJ Lanham, SM Provost, RR McDaniel Jr, and JA Pugh. 2014. "Improving outcomes of hospitalized patients: The physician relationships, improvising, and sense-making intervention protocol." *Implementation Science* 9 (1):171.

Leykum, LK, HJ Lanham, JA Pugh, M Parchman, RA Anderson, BF Crabtree, . . . RR McDaniel Jr. 2014. "Manifestations and implications of uncertainty for improving healthcare systems: An analysis of observational and interventional studies grounded in complexity science." *Implementation Science* 9 (1):165.

Lichtenstein, BB, and DA Plowman. 2009. "The leadership of emergence: A complex systems leadership theory of emergence at successive organizational levels." *The Leadership Quarterly* 20 (4):617–630. doi: 10.1016/j.leaqua.2009.04.006.

Mannion, R, and M Exworthy. 2017. "(Re) Making the procrustean bed? Standardization and customization as competing logics in healthcare." *International Journal of Health Policy and Management* 6 (6). doi: 10.15171/ijhpm.2017.35.

McAllister, C, LK Leykum, HJ Lanham, HS Reisinger, JL Kohn, RF Palmer, . . . RR McDaniel Jr. 2014. "Relationships within inpatient physician housestaff teams and their association with hospitalized patient outcomes." *Journal of Hospital Medicine* 9 (12):764–771.

McDaniel Jr, RR. 2007. "Management strategies for complex adaptive systems sensemaking, learning, and improvisation." *Performance Improvement Quarterly* 20 (2):21–41.

McKenna, K, LK Leykum, and RR McDaniel Jr. 2013. "The role of improvising in patient care." *Health Care Management Review* 38 (1):1–8.

Miller, JH, and SE Page. 2009. *Complex Adaptive Systems: An Introduction to Computational Models of Social Life. Vol. 17, Princeton Studies in Complexity*. Edited by SA Levin and SH Strogatz. Princeton: Princeton University Press.

Newman, M, A-L Barabási, and DJ Watts. 2006. *The Structure and Dynamics of Networks*. Princeton: Princeton University Press.

Weick, KE. 1993. "The collapse of sensemaking in organizations: The Mann gulch disaster." *Administrative Science Quarterly* 38 (4):628–652. doi: 10.2307/2393339.

Weick, KE. 1995. *Sensemaking in Organizations*. Vol. 3. Thousand Oaks: Sage.

Weick, KE. 2005. "Managing the unexpected: Complexity as distributed sensemaking." In *Uncertainty and Surprise in Complex Systems: Questions on Working with the Unexpected*, edited by R McDaniel and D Driebe. Berlin: Springer-Verlag.

Weick, KE, and KM Sutcliffe. 2003. "Hospitals as cultures of entrapment: A re-analysis of the Bristol royal infirmary." *California Management Review* 45 (2):73–84.

Weick, KE, KM Sutcliffe, and D Obstfeld. 2008. "Organizing for high reliability: Processes of collective mindfulness." *Crisis Management* 3 (1):81–123.

Zsambok, CE, and G Klein. 2014. *Naturalistic Decision Making*. New York: Psychology Press.

14 Simulation to solve health system problems

Mary D Patterson and Ellen S Deutsch

Introduction

The trauma team is called to the emergency department to care for a child injured in a motor vehicle crash. The team urgently inserts an emergency airway and ventilates the patient. A second child from the same motor vehicle crash arrives in the resuscitation bay. This patient also requires an emergency airway. However, as the team attempts to ventilate the patient, they find that there is insufficient oxygen pressure in the fixed oxygen tower to support simultaneous ventilation for both patients. Frantically, the team calls for portable oxygen tanks to ventilate both patients. Fortunately, these patients are 'simulators', but the safety hazard of inadequate oxygen pressure is real.

As a result of the simulation, the hazard is captured during the debriefing and the information is provided to clinical engineering to investigate and remediate. Two weeks later, the same simulation is repeated. This time, the oxygen pressure is sufficient to care for both patients simultaneously. All this occurs before the new hospital emergency department opens for real patients (Geis et al. 2011). The case presented demonstrates the importance of the observations that occur during in situ simulation (simulation that occurs in the clinical setting), but certainly no one would confuse this exercise with a clinical intervention or a randomized clinical trial.

Healthcare has an important and productive tradition of quantitative research, and blinded randomized controlled clinical trials (RCT) are thought of as the gold standard in medical research (Smith and Pell 2003; Speith et al. 2016). However, when one examines the history of healthcare, many of the theories that we now hold as dogma are based in astute observation and qualitative research. The germ theory of infectious disease famously arose from a series of observations by the nineteenth-century obstetrician Ignaz Semmelweis (and others) concerning the differences in the mortality rates between midwife-directed and surgeon-directed obstetric wards; the surgeons' ward had a substantially higher mortality rate. Sub-sequently, Semmelweis connected the process of surgeons moving directly from autopsies to the obstetric ward as the cause of "childbed fever" (Semmelweis 1847, 1983). Almost forty years later, Pasteur published a series of observations based on individual cases as the basis of the germ theory of infectious disease (Pasteur 1880, 2014).

For a variety of reasons, including ethical constraints, not all theories can be proven (or disproven) by quantitative research. The presumed necessity of using parachutes when skydiving despite a lack of RCTs proving their value provides a classic example (Smith and Pell 2003). The presumed necessity of using pulse oximetry in many healthcare settings provides a contemporary example. In 2011, the *New England Journal of Medicine* stated that "pulse oximetry is indicated in all clinical settings in which hypoxemia may occur" including operating rooms and other patient care units (Ortega et al. 2011). A Cochrane review published three years later and limited to RCTs found "no evidence that pulse oximetry affects the outcome of anaesthesia for patients" (Pedersen et al. 2014, 2). The ubiquitous adoption of pulse oximetry has occurred because it makes sense to expert providers, despite "the paucity of data that such devices improve outcome" (Jubran 2015, 6).

The strengths and limitations of qualitative research complement those of quantitative research (Anonymous 2017). Qualitative healthcare research can be used to explore beliefs, experiences, attitudes, behaviour and interactions and tackle questions about 'why and how' that may not be answerable with other techniques (Anonymous 2017; Elledge 2018; Pathak, Jena, and Kalra 2013). Simulation can provide unique and important resources for qualitative research. In particular, in situ simulation provides opportunities for observation of and by frontline healthcare professionals in circumstances that closely replicate both exceptional and everyday clinical work.

Applications

Simulation can be used for more than training technical and non-technical skills for individuals and teams. Simulation is a method for proactive assessment of threats, system capability and adaptive capacity as well as an activity that supports attitudinal and culture change.

In situ simulation, simulation that occurs in the clinical environment with frontline healthcare professionals, is particularly suited to a qualitative approach, and in fact research that utilizes in situ simulation often incorporates a primitive thematic analysis. Early studies incorporating in situ simulation often collected and categorized various types of safety threats in the clinical system based on observation and debriefing of participants. Though not specifically labeled as qualitative research, this work often incorporated participant observations from different microsystems and from different roles.

Threats identified during simulation are classified according to the type of threat and whether the threat is generalizable for more than one microsystem (Patterson et al. 2013; Wheeler et al. 2013). For example, during in situ simulations in a pediatric emergency department it was observed that medication dilution and administration for certain critical drugs was problematic. Based on these observations, in situ simulations for various pediatric critical care units were designed and implemented. Similar findings were identified in other patient care units, and resources to address this issue were deployed to all the affected clinical units. In this situation, knowledge gleaned from observation of in situ simulations combined with the domain knowledge of content experts facilitated the development of workable solutions without a formal clinical trial.

In a different application, in situ simulation can facilitate the development of an approach for rare, high-risk complex situations for which there will never be an ability to conduct a quantitative experiment. The separation of conjoined twins is a rare and high-risk procedure (Simpao et al. 2014). Clinical trials concerning this procedure are unlikely to ever exist given the rare occurrence of this condition. However, healthcare professionals can use simulation to begin to anticipate the complexity of this process and rehearse in a manner that surfaces specific hazards in order to minimize risk. Simulations of this procedure have and do occur (Simpao et al. 2014). It is likely that some of the data developed as a result of these simulations are potentially generalizable to other complex, infrequent and high-risk procedures that require the coordinated interaction of multiple specialties and multiple teams. The challenge then is the coding and analysis of the data gathered during these types of simulations.

The problem

Healthcare is a sociotechnical system. Though healthcare is delivered by teams, training often occurs in single discipline silos and in an environment very different from the one in which the healthcare team delivers care. As a result, individual healthcare professionals do not often have the opportunity to train with members of the healthcare team from different disciplines. There may be an absence of common behavioural and communication expectations. As well, the opportunity to identify and address hazards in the clinical environment is missed.

To this point, much of the qualitative research in simulation focuses on perceptions and perceived effectiveness of simulation-based training rather than the impact of simulation-based training on clinical care (Burke et al. 2017; Chancey et al. 2019; Sørensen et al. 2015). The reality of simulation training is that much of what is learned and described as an outcome occurs in a process that aligns with qualitative inquiry. However, the approach and the outcomes are rarely defined as qualitative research.

One of the strengths of simulation training is the opportunity to standardize the presentation of clinical situations in order to understand how different individuals and teams respond to clinical challenges in similar and dissimilar ways. The observed variation in response may reflect different kinds of knowledge, expertise and resources as well as varying perceptions of the clinical situation. These types of differences are not easily reduced to numbers and discrete solutions. How teams make decisions and move forward with various actions may be quite complex. Attempting to reduce these decisions and actions to numbers in predefined categories may be a disservice to the development of understanding. The nuanced and 'thick' understanding developed during debriefing has the potential to yield understanding of the knowledge and influences that inform decision-making and actions of individuals and team members. These may include knowledge unknown by one discipline that is well known to another discipline.

Qualitative examples of simulation debriefing studies and educational events

Debriefings following multidisciplinary simulations conducted on a simulated pediatric patient with an obstructed tracheostomy tube revealed that physicians and nurses had misperceptions of the others' skills with respect to the emergency management of tracheostomy tubes. Nurses were generally skilled in this domain but believed that all physicians had these skills as well and waited for an order to change the tracheostomy. Many physicians did not have these skills but also did not know that nurses were skilled in this area. Debriefing revealed this mismatch to each group. This insight was developed during repeated observations by the simulation facilitators and was subsequently shared as generalizable knowledge (Zaveri et al. 2018).

Simulation deliberately paired with a critical decision application of qualitative research methods was used to elicit differences in the ways that novice and expert acute care physicians approach an undifferentiated patient with possible sepsis (Patterson et al. 2016). The thematic analysis of these interviews was then used to develop simulations focused on novice physicians. The simulations were conducted using a 'freeze' or modified Situational Awareness Global Assessment Tool that provided the opportunity to ask what the physicians were paying attention to, what they believed was the cause of the patient's illness and what information they would be seeking in the next several minutes. The novice physicians' responses were also coded and analyzed (Geis et al. 2018). This particular project facilitated understanding of the differences in the ways that experts quickly recognize and manage sepsis. One key finding of this project is that experts tend to do more hypothesis testing than novice physicians. That is, experts will intervene with the explicit goal of understanding how a patient's response to specific clinical manoeuvers increases or lessens the likelihood of a particular diagnosis. This explicit use of qualitative methods for simulation research (aside from qualitative analysis of participants' impressions of simulation) is unusual. This may reflect the relative paucity of qualitative research expertise in the simulation community as well as a concern that there is a bias against publishing qualitative research.

Qualitative research has also been used to probe motivation to participate in simulation-based educational events. A series of one-to three-day simulation-based 'boot camps' has become popular as a method to provide intensive participatory education for novice residents and fellows in various disciplines. Having a sufficient number of expert faculty members provide individualized experiences is critical. Because faculty members are generally volunteers, and the boot camps occur on weekends, understanding factors that contribute to attracting and retaining faculty is important. A qualitative study addressing faculty motivation to participate in simulation-based boot camps identified the following themes:

> Enjoyment of teaching and camaraderie; benefits to residents, patients, and themselves; and opportunities to learn or improve their own patient care and teaching techniques emerged as leading elements of faculty motivation. Time away from work and family, as well as expense, were the major challenges.
>
> (Deutsch et al. 2013, 896)

Everyday clinical work

Hollnagel has proposed that the study of Everyday Clinical Work (ECW) requires a very different approach than that typically employed in quantitative clinical research. Hollnagel states:

> The study of ECW is done in order to understand clinical performance recognizing patterns in individual and collective behavior, to understand what determines the patterns and to ensure that everyday clinical work can be carried out in a manner that is both safe and efficient. This kind of research is by tradition qualitative.
>
> (Hollnagel 2015, 146)

Hollnagel describes a framework for this type of work: the Method, Classification Scheme and Model approach. In this approach the method is the way(s) in which data collection and data analysis occur. Simulation typically involves observation of the work performed during the simulated event. However, debriefing is an integral aspect of simulation and thus simulation data involves not only observations but also elicited information from the healthcare professionals who participate in simulation events (Hollnagel 2015). The boundaries of simulated events are typically related to the simulation event itself. However, as in situ simulation takes place in the clinical environment, it is often subject to the same dependencies as actual clinical work. Therefore, the simulation event may provoke exploration of the network of dependencies that are elicited during the simulation. This may occur through additional simulations or by querying healthcare professionals who are part of the organizational network.

Discussion

Many facilities have simulation resources; however, the potential for simulation to identify clinical hazards, enhance healthcare professionals' capabilities and improve system reliability is often underutilized or unrecognized. Simulation can surface both hazards and solutions, and provides a means to address many of the challenges of sociotechnical systems. Simulation provides integrated opportunities to probe the thought processes and actions of healthcare professionals and explore potential solutions to healthcare delivery challenges. Reflective debriefing, which is a key component of simulation, supports 'resonance' (Elledge 2018) by allowing exploration of key findings and verification of interpretations in conjunction with participants. We can describe two broad areas of observations that may emerge during debriefing and inform novel qualitative inquiry.

The first category is the interaction of individuals and the team with one another and the clinical system. This may include relational aspects and the adaptive capacity of individuals, teams and the system. Debriefings are typically rich sources of data around how individuals interact with one another and the influences and constraints on their communication and behaviour. Debriefing provides the opportunity to see oneself and one's colleagues in a different way. Knowledge of the 'other's' expertise is surfaced. The adaptive capacity (Nemeth et al. 2008) and the ways in which individual adaptation enables the team to adapt to predictable and unpredictable demands is explicitly defined. The importance of each individual's contributions to the team's performance is clarified.

The second category is the observations of actual threats and resources within the system. Most often these are described as safety threats, risks or constraints. However, supports or means to facilitate adaptation may also be observed, particularly if the debriefing is designed to elicit this type of information (Dieckmann et al. 2017). Often times, clinicians experience 'faint signals' concerning hazards. Alternatively, the clinicians may ask why a particular process is successful in one microsystem and not another. In either case, observations during in situ simulations and debriefing provide evidence (albeit not quantitative evidence) of risks to performance or conversely the elements that facilitate good performance.

Implications

The nature of in situ simulation lends itself to qualitative inquiry. Observations during the simulation inform the facilitator's exploration of why and how certain actions occur. Debriefing provides a 'built-in' opportunity to elicit this type of information from the clinical team members. In situ simulation provides a means to investigate weak signals, near misses and risk as well as to reliably support adaptive teams and good performance. The data gathered are not necessarily based on quantitative analysis but rather on the observations during the simulation as well as information elicited from healthcare professionals during debriefing. Though qualitative research has traditionally not been highly valued in medicine, which has tended to favour the RCT and other quantitatively oriented approaches, this type of investigation has the potential to be as valuable as early observations by Semmelweis and Pasteur.

Conclusion

Simulation is a powerful modality, frequently underutilized, that supports the development of resilient, adaptive performance. In addition, simulation, particularly debriefing, provides unique opportunities for qualitative research as both facilitators and participants are actively involved in analysis, as subjects and as collaborators providing complementary perspectives and providing rich, in-depth insights into what is happening in real world clinical practice.

References

Anonymous. 2017. "Understanding qualitative research in health care." *Drug and Therapeutics Bulletin* 55 (2):21.

Burke, RV, NE Demeter, CJ Goodhue, H Roesly, A Rake, LC Young, . . . JS Upperman. 2017. "Qualitative assessment of simulation-based training for pediatric trauma resuscitation." *Surgery* 161 (5):1357–1366.

Chancey, RJ, EM Sampayo, DS Lemke, and CB Doughty. 2019. "Learners' experiences during rapid cycle deliberate practice simulations: A qualitative analysis." *Simulation in Healthcare* 14 (1):18–28.

Deutsch, ES, A Orioles, K Kreicher, KM Malloy, and DL Rodgers. 2013. "A qualitative analysis of faculty motivation to participate in otolaryngology simulation boot camps." *The Laryngoscope* 123 (4):890–897.

Dieckmann, P, M Patterson, S Lahlou, J Mesman, P Nyström, and R Krage. 2017. "Variation and adaptation: Learning from success in patient safety-oriented simulation training." *Advances in Simulation* 2 (1):21.

Elledge, R. 2018. "Current thinking in medical education research: An overview." *British Journal of Oral and Maxillofacial Surgery* 56 (5):380–383.

Geis, GL, B Pio, TL Pendergrass, MR Moyer, and MD Patterson. 2011. "Simulation to assess the safety of new healthcare teams and new facilities." *Simulation in Healthcare* 6 (3):125–133.

Geis, GL, DS Wheeler, A Bunger, LG Militello, RG Taylor, JP Bauer, . . . MD Patterson. 2018. "A validation argument for a simulation-based training course centered on assessment, recognition, and early management of pediatric sepsis." *Simulation in Healthcare* 13 (1):16–26.

Hollnagel, E. 2015. "Looking for patterns in everyday clinical work." In *Resilient Health Care: The Resilience of Everyday Clinical Work*, edited by R Wears, E Hollnagel, and J Braithwaite. Vol. 2. Farnham: Ashgate Publishing, Ltd. 145–161.

Jubran, A. 2015. "Pulse oximetry." *Critical Care* 19 (272).

Nemeth, C, R Wears, D Woods, E Hollnagel, and R Cook. 2008. "Minding the gaps: Creating resilience in health care." In *Advances in Patient Safety: New Directions and Alternative Approaches. Vol. 3, Performance and Tools*, edited by K Henriksen, J Battles, M Keyes, and M Grady. Rockville: Agency for Healthcare Research and Quality.

Ortega, R, C Hansen, K Elterman, and A Woo. 2011. "Pulse oximetry." *New England Journal of Medicine* 364 (16):e33.

Pasteur, L. 1880, 2014. *On the Extension of the Germ Theory to the Etiology of Certain Common Diseases*. eBooks@Adelaide. Original edition, Comptes Rendus de l'Academie des Sciences.

Pathak, V, B Jena, and S Kalra. 2013. "Qualitative research." *Perspectives in Clinical Research* 4 (3):192.

Patterson, M, G Geis, R Falcone, T LeMaster, and R Wears. 2013. "In situ simulation: Detection of safety threats and teamwork training in a high risk emergency department." *BMJ Quality & Safety* 22 (6):468–477.

Patterson, M, L Militello, A Bunger, R Taylor, D Wheeler, G Klein, and G Geis. 2016. "Leveraging the critical decision method to develop simulation-based training for early recognition of sepsis." *Journal of Cognitive Engineering Decision Making* 10 (1):35–36.

Pedersen, T, A Nicholson, K Hovhannisyan, A Møller, A Smith, and S Lewis. 2014. "Pulse oximetry for perioperative monitoring." *Cochrane Database of Systematic Reviews* 3 (3).

Semmelweis, I. 1847, 1983. *The Etiology, Concept and Prophylaxis of Childhood Fever*. Translated by K Carter. Edited by K Carter. Madison: University of Wisconsin Press.

Simpao, A, R Wong, T Ferrera, H Hedrick, A Schwartz, T Snyder, . . . PJ Bailey. 2014. "From simulation to separation surgery: A tale of two twins." *Anesthesiology* 120 (1):110.

Smith, G, and J Pell. 2003. "Parachute use to prevent death and major trauma related to gravitational challenge: Systematic review of randomised controlled trials." *BMJ* 327 (7429):1459–1461.

Sørensen, J, L Nayne, H Martin, B Ottesen, C Albrecthsen, B Pederson, . . . C van der Vleuten. 2015. "Clarifying the learning experiences of healthcare professionals with in situ and off-site simulation-based medical education: A qualitative study." *BMJ Open* 5 (10):e008345.

Speith, P, A Kubasch, A Penzlin, BM-W Illigens, K Barlinn, and T Siepmann. 2016. "Randomized controlled trials – a matter of design." *Neuropsychiatric Disease and Treatment* 12:1341–1349.

Wheeler, D, G Geis, E Mack, T LeMaster, and M Patterson. 2013. "High-reliability emergency response teams in the hospital: Improving quality and safety using in situ simulation training." *BMJ Quality & Safety* 22 (6):507–514.

Zaveri, P, D Ren, M, R Batabyal, J Chamberlain, L Nicholson, R Sarnacki, . . . M Patterson. 2018. *Code Response Simulation Training to Improve Interprofessional Communication and Safety Behaviors*. Amsterdam, Netherlands: International Pediatric Simulation Symposium.

15 Cross-boundary teaming to establish resilience among isolated 'silos'

Kyota Nakamura, Shin Nakajima, Takeru Abe and Kazue Nakajima

Introduction

The healthcare field has been slow to employ implementation science ideas in improving care to patients. To enhance healthcare, the structure of the medical team by which staff cooperate, interact positively, and work dynamically must be clarified and generalized. Typically, team members with diverse backgrounds and specialties work successfully in a single department ('silo') of a healthcare institute. However, coordinated collaborations across multiple silos (multi-departments) often encounter difficulties, such as politically motivated 'us' and 'them' perspectives, even though such collaborations are imperative for safe care in clinical settings.

The difference between a single silo and multi-departments is attributed to team dynamics. Teams within a silo have daily interactions, whereas an improvised or *ad hoc* team needs to be established when multi-department collaboration is necessary, typically to deal with an atypical issue. Consequently, cross-boundary 'teaming' (the term used in this chapter to refer to teams working together), which is a common need in healthcare organizations, must overcome the shortcomings of siloed working patterns.

Although people in silos often understand the need for multi-department collaboration, it is often tactically difficult to obtain cooperation in actual practice. Successful cross-boundary teaming requires coordination to connect appropriate silos, but people within silos are busy, they have few incentives to collaborate more widely, and their attention is on their immediate work and contexts.

This chapter focuses on cross-boundary teaming and aims to clarify the factors and processes of coordination to establish effective cross-boundary teaming. Specifically, we review and analyze a Japanese case where multi-departments cooperated to resolve a difficult situation.

Context

Although medical care has advanced considerably in recent decades (Braithwaite et al. 2017), examinations and treatments involve risk, which is mitigated via risk management methods. For example, contrast-enhanced computed tomography

(CECT) examinations are routinely used to diagnose various diseases, but the radiographic contrast agent is a high-risk drug for anaphylaxis. Anaphylaxis is a rapidly progressing, severe allergic reaction, and asphyxia due to airway edema and severe hypotension can be fatal within 30 to 60 minutes. Fatal anaphylaxis is rare, but once it occurs, prompt systemic treatment is required (Kemp 2008).

Consider a case where CECT is performed in a computed tomography (CT) laboratory in the radiology department and where, in the case in question, the CT laboratory is not suited for systemic management of the patient due to space limitations and insufficient monitoring. On the other hand, the hospital itself is equipped with the appropriate resources such as staff with various specialties, ample space, and necessary equipment. In particular, a hybrid resuscitation room with a CT scan (Resus CT) is designed for on-site surgery and the space is equipped for systemic management with various medical devices such as monitors and ventilators. However, only emergency physicians use Resus CT as it was developed with financial support from the government for severe trauma care in the local area.

Considering the areas of expertise to treat anaphylactic shock, anaesthesiologists, emergency physicians, and cardiac surgeons all possess sufficient base-line knowledge and skills. Unlike emergency physicians who treat many cases of anaphylactic shock, however, anaesthesiologists and cardiac surgeons have limited experience. Emergency physicians usually perform anaesthesia management and medical treatment simultaneously for a severe trauma patient in Resus CT, but they focus on medical treatment. Although anaesthesiologists are the most qualified at anaesthesia and airway management, they do not oversee anaesthesia management outside the operating theatre (OT). The patient safety department serves as a hub for the in-hospital network, which manages safety issues across the hospital and knowledge about in-hospital resources.

Case study: scheduled CECT for a patient with a history of anaphylaxis to the radiographic contrast agent

Having established the context for this topic, we present a quadratic case study to exemplify the situation we have described. It begins with a radiographic procedure with a patient being transported to emergency care.

In the emergency department

An elderly male patient, who has a known allergy to the radiographic contrast agent, complained of a sudden onset of severe back pain and was transferred to the emergency department by paramedics. It was suspected that he had an acute aortic dissection. However, a CECT was necessary to determine the treatment pathway. During the CECT, he collapsed due to anaphylactic shock with severe laryngeal edema. The emergency department team struggled to secure his airway. Fortunately, the anaesthesiologist, who responded to a request for help, managed to intubate the patient. Eventually, the patient was diagnosed and underwent aortic stent graft placement.

Consultation from the cardiovascular team

One month later, the cardiovascular team thought that there was a risk of aorto-esophageal fistula due to an endoleak of the aortic stent graft. Another CECT was necessary to decide the treatment plan. The patient (and his family) wanted to undergo another CECT even if there was a risk of anaphylaxis. Weighing up the patient's preferences with the risk involved, the cardiovascular team consulted with the safety department, and a multidisciplinary team meeting was held to discuss how to proceed while minimizing risk.

Meeting and initial plan

Cardiovascular surgeons, ward nurses, including the chief nurse, intensivists, and patient safety officers participated in the first multidisciplinary team meeting. A CECT was planned after securing the patient's airway under general anaesthesia. An anaesthesiologist also consented to the treatment plan. Instead of using the CT laboratory, the procedure was to be performed in Resus CT, which would more easily provide systemic management. The multidisciplinary team was confident of this plan.

Barriers to coordination

Before the CECT was to begin, the multidisciplinary team asked a radiological technologist and the nurses in the department to use Resus CT. The radiological technologist responded that this would be difficult because Resus CT was designed for emergency severe trauma cases and not for scheduled inpatient examinations. The chief nurse also refused because there were no rules to manage anaesthetic drugs, including opioids, in Resus CT.

To address these problems, the multidisciplinary team asked an operating theatre pharmacist to use an anaesthesia cart in Resus CT because it contains many anaesthesia-related drugs and equipment. However, the OT pharmacist denied the request because there was a rule prohibiting the use of anaesthesia carts outside the OT.

True voices

To overcome this situation, the multidisciplinary team listened to everyone's opinions carefully. Then the team tried to identify the ostensible barriers and people's true concerns. These concerns could be divided into two areas: *responsibilities* and *irregularities* of the situation. The radiological technician was concerned about the liability of using Resus CT for a scheduled procedure in the event that an emergency severe trauma patient needed to be transferred. The nurses worried about increasing their workload related to this examination. In particular, management of anaesthetic drugs and chart recording are burdensome and are not part of their daily clinical work. The OT pharmacist was apprehensive about the consequences of using the anaesthesia cart outside the OT if an incident occurred with opioids or another anaesthetic drug as well as establishing a new precedent that transformed the current rules. After listening to each opinion and appreciating their real views, the team felt that these factors could be resolved through additional coordination efforts.

Second round coordination

After examining their beliefs, the team negotiated with the director of each department to coordinate roles and to secure the proper space and equipment.

The Director of Radiology supported the use of Resus CT if the Director of the Emergency Department concurred. The Director of the Emergency Department agreed to schedule this CECT examination on the condition that if another emergency patient was using Resus CT at the designated time, the procedure would be rescheduled. The Director of Pharmacy authorized use of an anaesthetic cart in Resus CT after considering the value of this examination plan. Similarly, the Director of Anaesthesia supported the plan.

Regarding the patient care plan, all parties agreed on the details of the plan and the specific roles assigned to staff. Emergency physicians were to manage the rescue treatment if the patient deteriorated due to anaphylaxis. An anaesthesiologist was to manage general anaesthesia, including medication management using an anaesthesia cart and recording a chart using the same protocols as those in the OT. Moreover, the nurses in Resus CT understood that their role would not deviate from their common clinical roles. Hence, consent and cooperation were obtained from all related departments.

Planned CECT examination

During the planned CECT, the patient developed anaphylaxis. Fortunately, the plan worked. The patient underwent an additional treatment for an endoleak of the aortic stent and left the hospital to recuperate at home.

Teaming in the healthcare setting

Even for routine illnesses, healthcare providers cannot simply use the same routine treatment for all patients. Currently, the patient population is aging, comorbidities are increasing, and medical care is becoming more complicated (Braithwaite et al. 2017). Consequently, safe medical care while embracing risk is necessary. When considering the provision of safe care for patients in this context, multidepartment cooperation is often needed. Teams must be built according to the challenges and goals on a case-by-case basis. These are variously known as ad hoc, transitory, or cross-boundary teams.

In normal operating environments, each specialist performs his or her role with high expertise in his or her silo. Silos with connections in daily clinical interactions routinely work as a team. However, healthcare is a '24/7', fast-paced operation, and it is not always possible to work with the same staff members and teamwork. In particular, if multi-department cooperation is needed to solve a problem, a mechanism to create an improvised team with first-time members or teams that usually do not collaborate should exist.

Edmondson and Harvey (2018) argued that knowledge diversity expands the range of views and ideas that teams can draw upon to innovate. For true innovation, people often need additional expertise and to work together across boundaries created by expertise, distance, and status. Edmondson and colleagues also indicated that cross-boundary teaming inside and across organizations has become a popular strategy for innovation and noted that an integration model was needed (Edmondson and Harvey 2018; Garvin, Edmondson, and Gino 2008; Nawaz et al. 2014; Edmondson 1999).

Previous studies such as a study investigating the Chilean mine accident (Rashid, Edmondson, and Leonard 2013) and the Lake Noma Medical City project case (Edmondson 2016) highlight the importance of high-level leadership for cross-boundary teaming. Innovation by cross-boundary teaming is a key factor to establishing a resilient system. Next we analyze how cooperation was performed in this case.

Comparison of a typical team and cross-boundary teaming

Like a sports team, strong teams, whether in one silo or multi-departments, have the following characteristics:

- Relative stability.
- Bounded group of individuals.
- Interdependent in achieving a shared goal.
- Typically practice together.

When building a multi-department team to solve a problem, the improvised team may contain first-time members. That is, new connections are required to solve a problem. Thus, each department must leave its silo, its routines, and its psychological safety.

In this case study, the cardiovascular team, anaesthesia department, emergency department, Resus CT nurses, pharmacy, and radiology collaborated. This teaming differs from a sports team. First, the members are not pre-identified. Second, there is no existing interdependence to achieve goals, and goal setting must be established. Third, the team does not practice regularly together. All these factors need to be managed.

How is a cross-boundary team built?

- Establish a network information hub and look beyond the silo.

Resources that are not in a silo's system can easily be overlooked. Additionally, it is difficult to evaluate skills and knowledge when working with new colleagues. Hence, available resources may not be considered. In this respect, proactively engaging colleagues in other departments may be important to fully consider all available resources.

In this case study, the cardiovascular team was initially considering the typical department protocol in the CT laboratory. That is, they viewed the situation from their normal clinic work perspective. Because people try to process information and events using what they know, the initial viewpoint is from the typical case. Hence, it is useful to find a team member who can act as a network information hub. This person not only knows where and what resources are available but also understands the movement of people in each silo. In this case study, a representative from the patient safety department, which oversees the entire hospital and understands the movement of people in each department, served as the hub and provided insight.

- Set goals and share.

The next step is to connect the necessary departments. Initially, a meeting was held where the cardiovascular team considered collaborating and discussed goal setting. As the cardiovascular team felt that using Resus CT for the patient under general anaesthesia was viable and realistic, team members were organized with confidence. Setting and sharing goals is a valuable step, especially when the team does not collaborate in daily clinical situations.

The collaborating team should set feasible goals. Consequently, it may be necessary to discuss a concrete tactical plan because the team's confidence in the plan is a driving force for coordination. After the initial goal and concrete tactics are set, it is important to repeat the evaluation and make corrections according to the situation. The results should be reshared with the team.

- Recognize the silos of related staff.

The original plan included the radiology department, Resus CT nurses, and anaesthesiologists. However, discussions revealed that the team should also include OT pharmacists and emergency physicians, demonstrating that tactical planning can identify key persons at the clinical field level. Although the opinions of key persons are very important, identifying and including the head of each silo may also be beneficial, as it was in our case.

- Arrange cross-boundary teaming.

We asked the radiology department, Resus CT nurses, and OT pharmacists for their cooperation. Although they understood the necessity of the plan, they could not immediately agree to cooperate. Each department had its own reasons for refusal. When arranging cross-boundary teaming, the typical response is that we agree with the plan but not the details. That is, each silo acknowledges the goal of the multi-department collaboration and understands the strategy but struggles in agreeing on the actual tactics for cooperation.

- Identify the real barriers by listening to the true voices of team members.

Are the reasons given by the radiology technicians, Resus CT nurses, and OT pharmacists the root cause? If the given reasons are considered as obstacles that can be addressed, then the implementation of the plan may seem feasible. What is the actual barrier? Will addressing the barrier lead to a real solution?

In a complex adaptive system, flexibility to respond to issues is important to engage team members. Hence, the team should include a key person from each silo. To identify the true voices of the clinical field, key persons should be involved in the discussions about the problem, resolution, and goal. These exchanges help all team members develop awareness, provide constructive opinions for problem-solving, and identify the root problems. Such interactions help key persons become effective team members.

Respond to true voices

We should examine and respond to the thoughts of each staff, and the beliefs that underpin their thoughts. The real voices of the frontline staff can be broadly divided into two categories: responsibility and workload.

In this case study, the concerns of the radiological technologist and OT pharmacist regarding responsibility were readily resolved by sharing the plan with the respective department director.

The issue with workload required more effort. One solution was to minimize the unconventional workload (both content and quantity) that may result from the situation. For example, it is usually a nurse's role to record a chart in Resus CT, but an anaesthesiologist was asked to record the chart in this case study. Anaesthesiologists do not feel burdened because anaesthesia recording is a routine task.

Additionally, if an anaesthesia cart is used to manage anaesthesia-related drugs, nurses might object as they are not involved in drug management. Managing the cart is part of the daily routine work of the anaesthesiologist. Since the preparation and post-treatment are part of normal routine of the OT pharmacist, the required workload is the same as daily operating.

On the other hand, from the anaesthesiologist's perspective, issues arise due to the location outside of OT and the patient's repeated history of anaphylaxis. Therefore, an emergency physician was asked to coordinate treatment if anaphylaxis developed. Emergency physicians use this space in daily practice and have abundant experience in treating anaphylaxis patients, whereas anaesthesiologists have knowledge and skills, but are not as experienced. These efforts secured psychological safety by eliminating concerns in response to the true voice of the staff.

Psychological safety

In Project Aristotle, Google researchers studied the secrets of effective teams (re:Work). The key to an effective team is working together. In order of importance, factors that influence team effectiveness are psychological safety, dependability, structure and clarity, meaning, and impact. Because frontline staff must step out of their silos in cross-boundary teaming, it may be more important to ensure psychological safety. When an irregular event occurs, psychological safety is achieved by sharing responsibility, easing workload, and adjusting the content of daily work as much as possible. Securing psychological safety of the frontline staff allows them to step beyond one silo, engage in a constructive discussion with team members in another, and have confidence in the plan made between silos, leading to a sense of control. Moreover, it should also create a positive loop that results in improvement.

Interpretation

Cross-boundary teaming is a key component to achieve many goals in healthcare. Figure 15.1 shows the conceptual scheme of problem-solving by independent silos

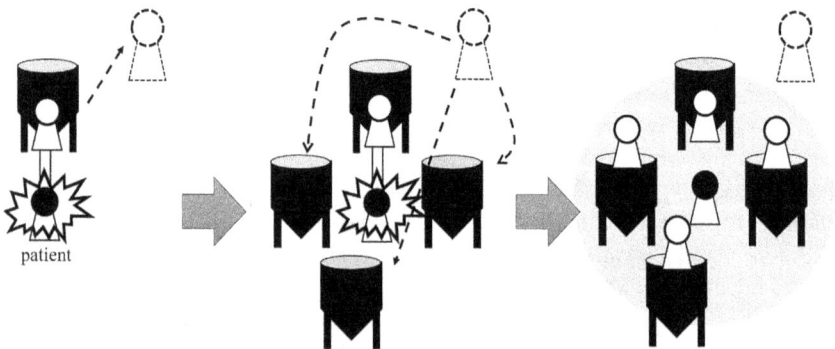

Figure 15.1 The formation of cross-boundary teams.

Source: Authors' own work.

and cross-boundary teaming, respectively. When a problem arises, it is useful to find a staff member who understands the movement of people working within each disciplinary 'silo' and where there are available resources to extend that work approach to a 'teaming' model of multi-departmental practice. The staff member can serve as a key element of the network hub and facilitate teaming. Next, the staff member calls on appropriate people from each silo to come together as a team, to voice their views of the problem in hand and to listen to one another. These exchanges help team members develop awareness of each other's work patterns while identifying barriers to teaming. Responding to the identified barriers to teaming guarantees better psychological safety for staff, and enables them to build new networks of silos, working according to a teaming model to solve healthcare problems.

Successful coordination for teaming involves several steps:

1   Identify a network hub person.
2   Share the overall purpose among the stakeholders and set the subsidiary goal.
3   Listen to the true voices of team members.
4   Identify the real barriers to achieve the goal.
5   Respond to those true voices.

These steps help establish a sense of control by broadening the authority of each silo, decentralizing responsibility, and reducing irregularities in the work. A sense of control by each member affirms psychological safety and flexibly broadens the boundaries between silos. In this way, the overall purpose of the teamwork can be achieved.

Conclusion

This case study and analysis clarified the coordination factors and processes that can help to build cross-boundary teaming. Cross-boundary teaming requires determining hub staff, pulling necessary resources from different silos, identifying true voices, and ensuring psychological safety.

References

Braithwaite, J, R Mannion, Y Matsuyama, P Shekelle, S Whittaker, and S Al-Adawi. 2017. *Health Systems Improvement Across the Globe: Success Stories from 60 Countries*. Boca Raton: CRC Press.

Edmondson, AC. 1999. "Psychological safety and learning behavior in work teams." *Administrative Science Quarterly* 44 (2):350–383.

Edmondson, AC. 2016. "Wicked problem solvers." *Harvard Business Review* 94 (6):52–59.

Edmondson, AC, and CF Harvey. 2018. "Cross-boundary teaming for innovation: Integrating research on teams and knowledge in organizations." *Human Resource Management Review* 28 (4):347–360.

156 *Kyota Nakamura et al.*

Garvin, DA, AC Edmondson, and F Gino. 2008. "Is yours a learning organization?" *Harvard Business Review* 86 (3):109.

Kemp, SF. 2008. "The post-anaphylaxis dilemma: How long is long enough to observe a patient after resolution of symptoms?" *Current Allergy and Asthma Reports* 8:45–48.

Nawaz, H, AC Edmondson, TH Tzeng, JK Saleh, KJ Bozic, and KJ Saleh. 2014. "Teaming: An approach to the growing complexities in health care." *The Journal of Bone and Joint Surgery* 96 (21):e184.

Rashid, F, AC Edmondson, and HB Leonard. 2013. "Leadership lessons from the Chilean mine rescue." *Harvard Business Review* 91 (7–8):113–119.

re:Work. "Guide: Understand team effectiveness." Google. Accessed August 2019. https://rework.withgoogle.com/print/guides/5721312655835136/.

16 "What on earth is going on and what should I do now?"

Sensemaking as a qualitative process

Kate Churruca, Louise A Ellis, Janet C Long and Jeffrey Braithwaite

Introduction

Sensemaking, quite literally, is about meaning-creation: the making of sense, particularly where things are complex, indeterminate, equivocal or uncertain. It involves perceiving, understanding and interpreting events and objects in our environment, but is also more than the sum of any one of these processes. Sensemaking is bound up with our actions, as our construction of meaning in any given situation becomes a basis for our actions and interactions with the world, in some ways, further determining that situation – a concept known as enactment. Such actions trigger new environmental stimuli as our movement through the world and experimentation with the objects within it (for example, picking them up or touching them) causes us to perceive new things, which may then lead to further sensemaking, and action.

Background

Organizational psychologist Karl Weick has had perhaps the biggest influence on the study of sensemaking in healthcare, although the development of the concept can be traced back to strands of work in ethnomethodology, cognitive and social psychology, and sociology (Weick 1995; Maitlis and Christianson 2014). Weick delineated seven properties of sensemaking (Table 16.1) and was concerned with how this process contributed to the functioning of organizations, not just in a business sense, but organizations as meaningful collective action among human beings (Weick 1993). He thus described how "once people begin to act (enactment), they generate tangible outcomes (cues) in some context (social), and this helps them discover (retrospect) what is occurring (ongoing), what needs to be explained (plausibility), and what should be done next (identity enhancement)" (1995, 55). In short, sensemaking is concerned with people asking (of themselves) "what on earth is going on?" and then when the answer comes to them, asking (of themselves) "what should I do now?" Then they plan to do it or talk to someone else to clarify their answers further.

Table 16.1 Seven properties of sensemaking

Property	Explanation
Grounded in identity construction	"How can I know what I think until I see what I say?" (Weick 1995, 18) Identity is always potentially multiple, and is therefore constituted in the process of interaction. Put another way, the self defines the situation, but the situation also defines the self. People project themselves into environments, but in doing so they also constitute their identities based on that situation. Indeed, sensemaking is triggered by situations that challenge our identities, and it typically functions to maintain a consistent, stable self-concept.
Retrospective	One can "know what they are doing only after they have done it" (Weick 1995, 24). In one sense, we experience the world as "pure duration", an ongoing and ephemeral stream of goings-on; however, whenever we sensemake we step outside this stream, giving our experiences the contours and boundaries of discrete events by putting our attention upon them. We are always looking back, retrospectively, in order to make sense of what we experience.
Enactive of sensible environments	People in part produce the environments they encounter; they are part of the environment and as they act upon it, they "create the materials that become the constraints and opportunities they face" (Weick 1995, 31). In acting on the environment, we produce stimuli that influence our sensemaking and then our subsequent actions (enactment).
Social	"Conduct is contingent on the conduct of others, whether those others are imagined or physically present" (Weick 1995, 39). Although sensemaking may involve shared meaning, this is not necessary; social sensemaking is also present as we coordinate our actions together with other people.
Ongoing	The flow of pure duration (of events, stimuli) is constant, and so in some ways, is sensemaking. At the same time, it involves looking back on and differentiating this experience into discrete events (retrospective). "To understand sensemaking is to be sensitive to the ways in which people chop moments out of continuous flows and extract cues from those moments" (Weick 1995, 43). This occurs in interruptions to the flow, where the environment changes in some way that we register, which stirs or arouses our emotions.
Focused on and by extracted cues	Environmental cues and changes prevail upon our senses, attracting our attention and interrupting the pure duration. People take pieces of these cues and signs, using them as reference points to construct their understanding of the greater whole event. "Extracted cues are simple, familiar structures that are seeds from which people develop a larger sense of what may be occurring" (Weick 1995, 50). Presumed ties between different cues are then made concrete by enacting them. However, what counts as a cue and how that cue is then interpreted are influenced by context.
Driven by plausibility rather than accuracy	"Accuracy is nice, but not necessary". It is more important that sensemaking is useful than truthful. An interpretation is useful insofar as it prompts action and provides a basis for further noticing of events in the environment and the extraction of cues. This leads to the embellishment and elaboration of sensemaking.

Source: Created by the authors from information in Weick, KE. 1995. *Sensemaking in Organizations.* Vol. 3. Thousand Oaks: Sage.

In perusing Table 16.1, we see that sensemaking involves an active role for the sense-maker in enacting his or her environment and constructing identity, that there are social aspects to sensemaking and that it is both ongoing and iterative. Many of these features call to mind the kinds of research questions and rich, interpretive analyses that are common in qualitative research, and particularly symbolic interactionism, and constructivist and constructionist approaches, which all focus on how meaning is constructed and the implications this has for action (Charmaz 2006).

Following Weick's work, diverging cognitive (that is, sensemaking taking place within the individual) and social (that is, sensemaking taking place between individuals) accounts of sensemaking have proliferated (Maitlis and Christianson 2014; Klein et al. 2007). What often results from this dichotomy is a focus on mental models, interpretations and frames (for individuals) versus communication, conversations and written texts (for groups). However, regardless of these somewhat different perspectives on the ontology of sensemaking, the primacy of qualitative methods in studying the process is clear. Indeed, Weick himself suggested that

> people who study sensemaking oscillate ontologically because that is what helps them understand the actions of people in everyday life who could care less about ontology . . . over time people will act like interpretivists, functionalists, radical humanists, and radical structuralists.

> (1995, 35)

Methods for studying sensemaking

Sensemaking can be studied using a range of qualitative, quantitative and mixed methods. However, as we have suggested, the majority of the empirical research on sensemaking in organizations has made use of qualitative methods, because they are "well-suited to the study of dynamic processes, especially where these processes are constituted of individuals' interpretations" (Maitlis 2005, 23). Hence, interviews, ethnographic data and organizational documents are often utilized for studying sensemaking. Interviews, in particular, allow us an opportunity to elicit people's retrospective sensemaking because most interviews are built in this way; they involve individuals unpicking a course of action by starting from the outcome, using this to create a story that is meaningful and internally consistent, and narrating that story. The account told in an interview is removed from the outcome and course of action that 'led' to it and is potentially exposed to further embellishment and reframing.

Observations, unlike interviews, are an important method for studying sensemaking in real time (Maitlis and Christianson 2014). During observations, capturing some of the more fine-grained aspects of sensemaking requires that we remain prepared at all times. It is not possible to predict the unexpected, and yet such situations are most likely to trigger sensemaking in individuals; this makes it difficult to "find people in the act of coping with disconfirmations that catch them unawares" (Weick, Sutcliffe, and Obstfeld 2005, 415). In this vein, Weick writes how:

> Sensemaking tends to be swift, which means we are more likely to see products than processes. To counteract this, we need to watch how people deal with prolonged puzzles that defy sensemaking, puzzles such as paradoxes, dilemmas, and inconceivable events. We also need to pay close attention to ways people notice, extract cues, and embellish that which they extract.
>
> (Weick 1995, 49)

The ephemeral nature of sensemaking processes, therefore, makes attempts to study them in situ within healthcare challenging, but nevertheless worthwhile. If observations are undertaken, extended time in the setting, through case study or ethnographic design, is warranted. Adding to this, and the ethnographic researcher's fieldnotes, the use of visual and audio recordings of events may facilitate the apprehension of sensemaking processes as they unfold (Mesman 2011). A final point to consider is the meta-issue of how the researcher's own sensemaking comes into play throughout the process of collection, analysis and interpretation of data. Similar to our interview participants, with increasing levels of extrapolation and the passage of time, we researchers are often more able to give our findings coherency and some level of rationality (Magolda 2000), but this is also something of which we should be reflexively sceptical. After all, researchers are sensemaking about sensemaking, when studying sensemaking processes.

Sensemaking in healthcare

Sensemaking theories have permeated both the conceptual and empirical analyses of healthcare settings over the past two decades (Leykum et al. 2015; Martin 2011). Having delineated the features of sensemaking and having made brief comments on some of the methods of studying it, we now consider three reasons for its applicability in healthcare.

First, sensemaking is considered particularly important on occasions of uncertainty and complexity, where our expectations may be thwarted (Klein et al. 2007). Healthcare settings are saturated with varying types of uncertainty (Pomare et al. 2019), as well as sharing features with other complex systems, meaning they are difficult to predict and events seem to emerge, often unexpectedly, from localized interactions (Braithwaite et al. 2017).

Second, healthcare delivery is typically a fast-paced and time-pressured environment (Braithwaite et al. 2018); action is always required before all the facts can possibly be gathered. This returns us to the point about plausibility over accuracy, a core feature of sensemaking: "It is more crucial to get some interpretation to start with than to postpone action until 'the' interpretation surfaces" (Weick 1995, 57).

Third, sensemaking is a basis for organizing, the collective action among human beings in institutions such as hospitals. Such collective action is paramount in the delivery of care to patients, where care coordination, integration and interprofessional collaboration must occur at multiple levels (Powell Davies et al. 2008; Reeves and Lewin 2004; Braithwaite et al. 2012a, 2012b). It involves people 'getting on the same page', which entails some measure of shared sensemaking.

This is not to say that the act of sensemaking is a purely positive force in clinical practice; rather that the conditions of work in healthcare settings make it commonplace and necessary, and therefore something that we should study and understand in the healthcare context. Indeed, Weick and Sutcliffe (2003), analyzing the organizational factors involved in a high number of deaths among paediatric cardiac surgery patients, noted how sensemaking around behavioural commitment led surgeons to a reading of their performance as 'doing their best' with complex cases, instead of the alternative understanding that they were doing poorly and needed to improve.

Studies of sensemaking in healthcare

The number of studies on sensemaking in healthcare has grown exponentially over the past few decades (see Figure 16.1). They have focused on issues of organizational change, clinical uncertainty and decision-making, patient safety and managerial practice (Ericson 2001; Dowding et al. 2016; Blatt et al. 2006; Checkland et al. 2013). They have been conducted in a range of different healthcare

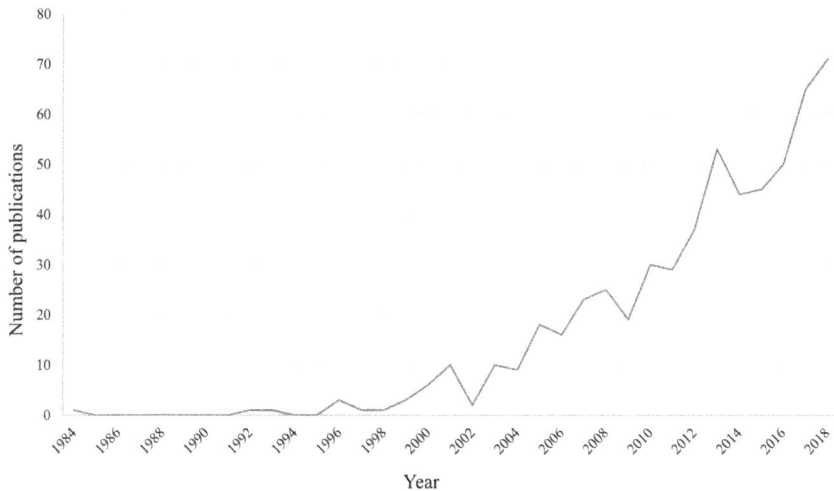

Figure 16.1 Publications on sensemaking in healthcare.

Source: Authors' charting of Scopus data. Based on search conducted on 15 May 2019 using search string: (TITLE-ABS-KEY (healthcare OR "health care" OR "health-care" OR "hospital" OR "health facilit*" OR "acute care" OR "health organi*" OR "primary care" OR "general practice" OR "aged care" OR "nurs* home" OR "clinic*" OR "medic*") AND TITLE-ABS-KEY ("sensemaking" OR "sense making" OR "sense-making")).

settings – including primary care facilities, hospitals and nursing homes – and involved stakeholders such as nurses, doctors, paramedics, general practitioners, consumers, IT staff and managers (Aanestad and Jensen 2016; Apker 2004; Checkland et al. 2009). In the remainder of this chapter, we discuss a selection of these studies, chosen for consideration because they are exemplars of a range of qualitative methods used for studying sensemaking, while covering a multitude of issues, settings and participants in healthcare.

Organizational change

Organizational change requires that individuals adapt their behaviour, but this in turn inevitably requires reinterpretation of both organizational and individual identity (Apker 2004). Sensemaking provides a useful framework for understanding both processes of organizational change and potential resistance to it (Checkland et al. 2009). Hultin and Mähring (2017) conducted a study of organizational change through the implementation of Lean manufacturing principles, which involves process improvement through streamlining, and the elimination of various forms of 'waste'. The study conducted in a Swedish emergency department (ED) took a radically social view of sensemaking in drawing upon a relational ontology. The researchers used an ethnographic design, which included interviews with, and observations of, nurses, doctors, the unit manager and the improvement team, in addition to analysis of archival data. Sensemaking was not only part of the researchers' conceptual framework but utilized in data analysis, as they grouped extracts together based on descriptions of enactments by the same subject groups (e.g., flow nurses responsible for ensuring patient pathways are streamlined and senior specialists). Their approach to sensemaking was based in a material-discursive epistemology, focusing on the physical environment of sensemaking (material) while decentralizing the subject (discursive). In this way, the approach suggests that actions create subject positions through which certain types of sense can be made, rather than implying the agency of the sense-maker. For example, the flow nurse, by virtue of her position within the "flow of agency" sensed the practice of sending patients to other wards before diagnosing them as the most appropriate (2017, 580). This approach to sensemaking also allowed Hultin and Mähring (2017) to demonstrate the important role of artefacts and materiality in producing particular types of sense within the ED. The flow board, a large electronic board visible in the ED which visualizes patient flow compared to standards set for optimal patient flow (i.e., for admissions, waiting times etc.), was a powerful influence on sensemaking in this hospital. It constituted what was previously an "interpenetrating flow of medical work" in examining patients and admitting them to beds in the hospital, as something that could be sectioned, quantified and measured to assess performance (Hultin and Mähring 2017, 587).

Safety

Sensemaking is important to the enactment of safety among frontline staff, as well as to a broader appreciation of how things go right or wrong in healthcare

(Sheps et al. 2015). A study of sensemaking in operating theatres by Rosness et al. (2016) uniquely focused on situations previously characterized by Weick as "non-events" (Weick 1987), in other words when operations proceeded smoothly in contrast to focusing on adverse events. The authors' perspective, as distinct from Weick's, recognized that operations that pass smoothly during surgical procedures were not associated with few things happening, but rather "many things happening" (Rosness et al. 2016, 54). According to Weick, organizational sensemaking is retrospective in that we make sense of our actions and experiences *after* they occur. However, Rosness et al.'s (2016) work suggests that prospective sense-making contributes to the safe and efficient completion of surgical procedures: staff create "plausible projections" of what might occur during surgery and plan *preemptively* to manage these possibilities. Their study was based on direct observations, semi-structured interviews and informal conversations with personnel (e.g., surgeon, anaesthetic nurses) involved in the operations. However, their focus on prospective sensemaking processes was not part of the initial framing of the study but rather derived following an analysis of their initial findings. In this way, their research approach was highly iterative and properly characterized as abductive in that the researchers started with a set of observations and tried out various interpretative frames, leading them to develop their hypothesis. The researchers then returned to the surgical ward to test their hypothesis and identify the characteristics of prospective sensemaking and its relation to safe and efficient performance.

Clinical decision-making

Studies of sensemaking in the clinical realm shed light on common clinical practices. Barley and colleagues (Barley et al. 2008) examined the different sources of knowledge that psychiatrists draw upon to make clinical decisions using semi-structured interviews. In their study of sensemaking around prescribing choices for people with schizophrenia they identified a complex mix of four types of knowledge contributing to the process: acquired, interpreted, individual experience and contextual. Clinical guidelines, in contrast to the expectations of their creators, informed only a small part of the decision. In another study, Nixon and Vendelo (2016) studied general practitioners' (GPs) sensemaking around the issue of statin prescription and discontinuation using interviews, document analyses and observations. GPs they interviewed could give examples of how they decided to prescribe statins; they weighed risk factors such as diabetes and smoking to inform their decision, factoring in that statins were a well-proven medication, inexpensive and largely safe. When it came to clinical decision-making around *discontinuation* of statins it was quite different. None of the GPs discussed patient perspectives such as a patient's preference to not take medications, suggesting these issues were not part of their sensemaking. More tellingly, none of the GPs could give an example of a situation where they discussed and recommended discontinuation. The authors concluded from the document analysis of the guidelines that the GPs were influenced strongly by the implied and overt messages embedded in the guidelines which communicated that discontinuation was not desirable or appropriate behaviour.

Conclusion

Sensemaking is the ongoing interpretation and enactment of the complex and dynamic environments in which we work and live. This chapter has examined sensemaking as an analytical framework, one particularly well suited to use with qualitative methods. Focusing largely on the seminal work of Weick, and building on empirical knowledge in studies in healthcare, we have described the seven aspects of sensemaking and considered the methods used for studying it. We have then considered how the concept has been most promisingly applied to healthcare in broad areas like organizational change, safety and clinical decision-making. As researchers and authors, we too have been sensemaking – but in our case, we have been sensemaking about sensemaking, trying to understand what on earth is going on and what we should do next.

References

Aanestad, M, and TB Jensen. 2016. "Collective mindfulness in post-implementation IS adaptation processes." *Information and Organization* 26 (1):13–27.

Apker, J. 2004. "Sensemaking of change in the managed care era: A case of hospital-based nurses." *Journal of Organizational Change Management* 17 (2):211–227.

Barley, M, C Pope, R Chilvers, A Sipos, and G Harrison. 2008. "Guidelines or mindlines? A qualitative study exploring what knowledge informs psychiatrists decisions about antipsychotic prescribing." *Journal of Mental Health* 17 (1):9–17.

Blatt, R, MK Christianson, KM Sutcliffe, and MM Rosenthal. 2006. "A sensemaking lens on reliability." *Journal of Organizational Behavior: The International Journal of Industrial, Occupational and Organizational Psychology and Behavior* 27 (7):897–917.

Braithwaite, J, K Churruca, LA Ellis, J Long, R Clay-Williams, N Damen, . . . K Ludlow. 2017. *Complexity Science in Healthcare – Aspirations, Approaches, Applications and Accomplishments: A White Paper.* Sydney, Australia: Australian Institute of Health Innovation, Macquarie University.

Braithwaite, J, LA Ellis, K Churruca, and JC Long. 2018. "The goldilocks effect: The rhythms and pace of hospital life." *BMC Health Services Research* 18 (1):529.

Braithwaite, J, M Westbrook, P Nugus, D Greenfield, J Travaglia, W Runciman, . . . J Westbrook. 2012a. "Continuing differences between health professions' attitudes: The saga of accomplishing systems-wide interprofessionalism." *International Journal for Quality in Health Care* 25 (1):8–15.

Braithwaite, J, M Westbrook, P Nugus, D Greenfield, J Travaglia, W Runciman, . . . J Westbrook. 2012b. "A four-year, systems-wide intervention promoting interprofessional collaboration." *BMC Health Services Research* 12 (1):99.

Charmaz, K. 2006. *Constructing Grounded Theory: A Practical Guide Through Qualitative Analysis.* London: Sage.

Checkland, K, A Coleman, S Harrison, and U Hiroeh. 2009. " 'We can't get anything done because . . . ': Making sense of 'barriers' to practice-based commissioning." *Journal of Health Services Research & Policy* 14 (1):20–26.

Checkland, K, S Harrison, S Snow, A Coleman, and I McDermott. 2013. "Understanding the work done by NHS commissioning managers: An exploration of the microprocesses underlying day-to-day sensemaking in UK primary care organisations." *Journal of Health Organization and Management* 27 (2):149–170.

Dowding, D, V Lichtner, N Allcock, M Briggs, K James, J Keady, . . . S José Closs. 2016. "Using sense-making theory to aid understanding of the recognition, assessment and management of pain in patients with dementia in acute hospital settings." *International Journal of Nursing Studies* 53:152–162.

Ericson, T. 2001. "Sensemaking in organisations – Towards a conceptual framework for understanding strategic change." *Scandinavian Journal of Management* 17 (1):109–131.

Hultin, L, and M Mähring. 2017. "How practice makes sense in healthcare operations: Studying sensemaking as performative, material-discursive practice." *Human Relations* 70 (5):566–593.

Klein, G, JK Phillips, EL Rall, and DA Peluso. 2007. "A data – frame theory of sensemaking." In *Expertise Out of Context: Proceedings of the Sixth International Conference on Naturalistic Decision Making*, edited by RR Hoffman. New York: Lawrence Erlbaum Associates. 113–155.

Leykum, LK, H Chesser, HJ Lanham, P Carla, R Palmer, T Ratcliffe, . . . JA Pugh. 2015. "The association between sensemaking during physician team rounds and hospitalized patients' outcomes." *Journal of General Internal Medicine* 30 (12):1821–1827.

Magolda, PM. 2000. "Accessing, waiting, plunging in, wondering, and writing: Retrospective sense-making of fieldwork." *Field Methods* 12 (3):209–234.

Maitlis, S. 2005. "The social processes of organizational sensemaking." *Academy of Management Journal* 48 (1):21–49.

Maitlis, S, and M Christianson. 2014. "Sensemaking in organizations: Taking stock and moving forward." *The Academy of Management Annals* 8 (1):57–125.

Martin, C. 2011. "Distortions, belief and sense making in complex adaptive systems for health." *Journal of Evaluation in Clinical Practice* 17 (2):387–388.

Mesman, J. 2011. "Resources of strength: An exnovation of hidden competences to preserve patient safety." In *A Socio-Cultural Perspective on Patient Safety*, edited by J Waring and E Rowley. Farnham: CRC Press.

Nixon, MS, and MT Vendelo. 2016. "General practitioners' decisions about discontinuation of medication: An explorative study." *J Health Organ Manag* 30 (4):565–580.

Pomare, C, K Churruca, LA Ellis, JC Long, and J Braithwaite. 2019. "A revised model of uncertainty in complex healthcare settings: A scoping review." *Journal of Evaluation in Clinical Practice* 25 (2):176–182.

Powell Davies, G, AM Williams, K Larsen, D Perkins, M Roland, and MF Harris. 2008. "Coordinating primary health care: An analysis of the outcomes of a systematic review." *Medical Journal of Australia* 188:S65–S68.

Reeves, S, and S Lewin. 2004. "Interprofessional collaboration in the hospital: Strategies and meanings." *Journal of Health Services Research & Policy* 9 (4):218–225.

Rosness, R, TE Evjemo, T Haavik, and I Wærø. 2016. "Prospective sensemaking in the operating theatre." *Cognition, Technology & Work* 18 (1):53–69.

Sheps, S, K Cardiff, R Pelletier, and R Robson. 2015. "Revealing resilience through critical incident narratives: A way to move from safety-I to safety-II." In *Resilient Health Care: The Resilience of Everyday Clinical Work. Vol. III, Resilient Health Care*, edited by RL Wears, E Hollnagel, and J Braithwaite. Farnham: Ashgate Publishing, Ltd. 189–206.

Weick, KE. 1987. "Organizational culture as a source of high reliability." *California Management Review* 29 (2):112–127.

Weick, KE. 1993. "The collapse of sensemaking in organizations: The Mann Gulch disaster." *Administrative Science Quarterly* 38 (4):628–652.

Weick, KE. 1995. *Sensemaking in Organizations*. Vol. 3. Thousand Oaks: Sage.

Weick, KE, and KM Sutcliffe. 2003. "Hospitals as cultures of entrapment: A re-analysis of the Bristol Royal Infirmary." *California Management Review* 45 (2):73–84.

Weick, KE, KM Sutcliffe, and D Obstfeld. 2005. "Organizing and the process of sensemaking." *Organization Science* 16 (4):409–421.

17 Deep inside the genomics revolution

On the frontlines of care

Stephanie Best, Janet C Long, Elise McPherson, Natalie Taylor and Jeffrey Braithwaite

Introduction

Assembling a person's entire human genetic information, their genome, through what is known as genomics, offers a revolutionary approach to healthcare provision, including diagnosis and treatment options. Genomics is a transformative innovation that will impact healthcare provision with implications across all life stages, body systems and conditions. Evidence of its impact on healthcare is emerging from the work of early adopters (Biesecker and Green 2014; Stark et al. 2017; Walsh et al. 2017). Genomics is a complex, multi-stage process that requires specialist knowledge, and the pooling of expertise across different laboratory scientists, healthcare professions and settings, with an overarching, deep concern about the uncertainty of genetic results in terms of, for example, the management of expectations (such as those of clinicians and patients), indicating a multitude of ethical challenges.

The research and linked qualitative methods described in this chapter were conducted as part of the Australian Genomic Health Alliance (hereafter known as Australian Genomics). Australian Genomics secured a record AUS$25 million funding from the Australian National Health and Medical Research Council's targeted call for grants in 2015. Australian Genomics is made up of over 80 partner organizations from across Australia, including medical researchers, biostatisticians, clinicians, consumers, health economists and health services researchers (Australian Genomic Health Alliance 2018). Australian Genomics includes close partnerships with state-based genomic alliances including Melbourne Genomics. The stated objective of Australian Genomics is to introduce clinical genomics into routine patient care throughout Australia using an accumulation of clinical utility and cost-effectiveness evidence across a wide range of conditions.

The problem in a nutshell

While evidence of clinical benefit is growing from both Australian work and the broader global effort in genomic research, the shift from laboratory to clinical practice has been slow. Around the turn of the century, Korf (2002, 10s) noted that with the onset of genome sequencing "genetics has become the driving force in medical research and is now poised for integration into medical practice". A decade and a half later, this implementation has yet to be fully realized.

The challenge and task ahead

The challenge, common to many radical innovations, is making things work in the real world: getting technology into practice. In this case, for genomics, the specific task is to enable the move from the laboratory into the clinic (Wolf et al. 2018). At the frontline of healthcare, the genomic translation hurdles that stand out are twofold: 1) translation from laboratory findings to research-based clinical practice and 2) transition from a research-based clinical practice to routine clinical care (Figure 17.1). All too often there is a focus on the basic research and a failure to address the translational gap, resulting in what might be perceived as the misappropriation of funding and a lack of improved care for patients (Chalmers and Glasziou 2009).

Pathways to addressing the problem

As with any complex, real world problem, tackling the challenges inherent in implementing genomics requires a multi-faceted approach. Working with Australian Genomics to examine these issues we selected a variety of qualitative methods to identify ways in which to facilitate translation, through: a) 'process mapping' to enable us to visually describe workflow in genetic clinics; b) key messages from surveys, to establish the Australian Genomics community's perception of the focus of Australian Genomics; and c) interviews with genomics specialists and decision makers, to identify barriers and enablers to implementation of genomics into the clinical setting. Each of these approaches provided us with a different lens with which to investigate implementation challenges, and each approach had its incumbent advantages and disadvantages. For example, time for analysis and participant engagement varies dramatically with each method and in different settings.

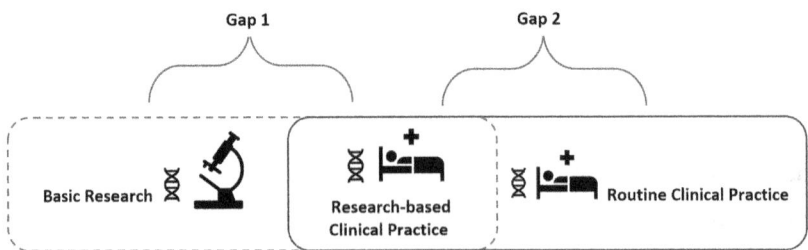

Figure 17.1 The phases and gaps in moving genomics basic research into practice.
Source: Authors' own work.

Methods

Genomic clinics are different to the traditional clinics due to their multistaged processes, requiring a range of specialists' knowledge across multiple disciplines and the current, inherent uncertainty of results. Clinical genomics is relevant to many different clinical specialities such as the field of renal medicine. A way of understanding the complexity of multistaged processes, mixed specialist group involvement and uncertain results in fields like renal genomics is by using qualitative research methods. Here we draw on examples from three different studies commissioned by Australian Genomics undertaken by our team using three different qualitative methods to discuss the use and value of qualitative methods in this domain (see Table 17.1).

Qualitative data were drawn from a large online survey of all members of Australian Genomics (n=225). The predominantly quantitative survey examined collaborative relationships in genomics, in order to map the emerging 'learning community' (Long et al. 2019). Participants were medical and genetic specialists, medical scientists, community advisors and researchers. Qualitative data were included in the survey, and were drawn from free text responses within a question which asked about respondents'

Table 17.1 Summary of the three qualitative methods used for researching the implementation of genomics in clinical practice

	Survey	Interviews	Process maps
Source of data	Free text qualitative responses in larger survey.	Interviews with key people (Taylor et al. 2019).	Senior informants.
Number of participants	225 out of a total of 384 members of Australian Genomics.	37 members of Australian Genomics or Melbourne Genomics.	Five senior members of a Flagship of Australian Genomics.
Characteristics of participants	Clinicians, genetic specialists, project officers, medical scientists, governing body members, consumer advisors, researchers.	Service-level decision makers and non-genomic medical specialists.	Medical specialists, clinical geneticists.
Analysis methods	Coding in NVivo to find themes and narratives around translation of biomedical research findings into clinical practice.	Capability, Opportunity, and Motivation Behaviour model (Michie, Van Stralen, and West 2011).	Process maps developed from informants' descriptions of workflow.

Source: Authors' own work.

understanding of the aims of Australian Genomics (stated on the collaboration's website as integrating genomics into routine practice in Australian healthcare; Australian Genomic Health Alliance 2018). Qualitative data also provided details of survey respondents' personal roles in achieving these aims. The qualitative questions were of particular interest, as within this collaborative endeavour, a shared understanding of purpose and perception of personal roles and accountability was seen as vital to explaining the success or otherwise of genomic integration into routine clinical practice.

Interviews were undertaken with 37 people working with either Australian Genomics or Melbourne Genomics. The interview format was semi-structured, and interviews took around 40 minutes to one hour to conduct and were mainly face-to-face (with four conducted either by telephone or via videoconference). All potential interviewees identified by the programme leads for Melbourne Genomics and Australian Genomics were invited to be interviewed (with a fall out rate of 37/62). The interview guides were informed by evidence-based frameworks of behaviour change and implementation. The aim was to identify challenges to implementing genomics in clinical practice according to behaviour change and other characteristics.

Process maps, which are a graphic representation of clinical processes and places where decisions are made, were generated from interviews with five senior clinicians from the five, state-based renal genetics clinics, working as the KidGen collaborative (a collaboration between clinical, diagnostic and research teams across Australia). KidGen operates a series of flagships under the auspices of Australian Genomics and had identified Flagship Leads in these clinics. The clinics were all part of a research-based, clinical renal genetics programme that shared the common aim of wishing to better understand the causes of inherited kidney disease using multidisciplinary teams in the clinical setting. Process mapping was undertaken to better understand why the clinics worked according to a range of different activities and clinical outcomes. The process maps, showing the workflow from the time a patient is referred to their discharge, were created with the clinicians to identify any process differences. The maps were initially drawn using Microsoft PowerPoint (V16.2). The structure of the maps provided a useful framework for discussion. They were then shown to participants to check for accuracy prompting reflection on processes and leading to further discussion. Maps were refined as necessary in response to feedback.

As with all research methods there are benefits and limitations to their in-context applicability, and this holds true for the three qualitative approaches used in the case study which are highlighted in Table 17.1, when applied to the specific context of Australian Genomics. The section that follows, and Table 17.2, outline a number of considerations for researchers to think through before applying these methods.

Table 17.2 Summary of considerations around the use of qualitative methods in the context of genomics research

	Survey: Free text responses	Interview: Semi-structured	Process map: Discussion and agreement
Potential size of population engaged	Large. Invitations to participate can be extended to extensive numbers of potential participants across population groups, cohorts and participant disciplines/cultural groups.	Limited, according to the resources available for undertaking interviews (face-to-face or through telephone/video calls).	Limited to a particular context.
Role of researcher	To design, format, pilot and distribute a survey, or specific survey questions that will accurately reflect the population being sampled.	To develop the interview schedule in order to draw out the participants' experiences.	To draw out the participants' views of activities and priorities.
Time commitment to set up and run	Medium. Online surveys involve less time in distribution and data collection.	Activity either side of data collection is time consuming (such as the organization of interviews and data management). The time commitment for interviewing varies according to the style and the length of the interview.	Medium. A basic understanding of the process under scrutiny is needed. Identification of appropriate key informants.
Time commitment for analysis	Small to medium, depending on the nature of the data. Online survey platforms allow data downloads directly to analysis software, saving transcription time and reducing error.	Large. Analyzing interviews is an iterative, in-depth process, requiring consultation with others and extensive periods of time investigating meaning and interpreting others' understanding of meaning-making.	Medium. A process map often goes through multiple iterations before participants agree it is accurate.
Purpose	To get answers from a particular population or representative sample of a population.	To learn from the participants who have experience in the field.	To show activities, interactions, interdependencies. May reveal a discrepancy between what work is imagined and the actual work taking place.

Source: Authors' own work.

Considerations for the use of qualitative methods in genomic investigation

Traditionally seen as a quantitative resource, surveys can be harnessed for qualitative research using questions that offer a free text response. This approach has the advantage of reaching a large population group and is relatively quick to set up and run. However, there is no opportunity to interrogate the responses further within the same survey (although other qualitative methods can be employed to collect secondary data to address this), to identify additional nuance and to examine any misunderstandings derived from survey questions.

By contrast, interviews take longer to organize and conduct, and apply to a smaller population group, with data management adding to the workload. However, they facilitate an interactive approach and where semi-structured interviews are used (as in Table 17.1) the study design can be usefully flexible to accommodate new knowledge. Learning can be iterative, with researcher knowledge and understanding developing from interview to interview.

The discussions held around process mapping is one of the valuable aspects of this approach, as participants gain insight into the complexities of their work experiences and a greater appreciation of 'up-stream' and 'down-stream' processes being carried out by others. For example, the complexity of organizing a multidisciplinary clinic may not be apparent to the clinician who is inviting others to attend. In addition, the structured presentation of the maps makes it easier for the researcher and participants to target points for particular attention, audit or quality improvement. As outlined in Table 17.2, process mapping is a relatively simple approach that requires no equipment or complex analysis. However, it does take time to engage key stakeholders, and time to ensure the process is fully understood by the researcher, so they not only acquire a sufficient depth of understanding but capture all of the complexities of the process under discussion.

Findings

Each of the three methods that were used when researching the implementation of clinical genomics generated different findings. Here we provide some of the highlights.

The free text survey answers around respondents' personal roles in achieving the aim of implementing genomics into routine care elicited some diverse and rich data. As well as the expected responses of: "My role is to lead/coordinate/facilitate/support/advocate" or "I am a member of the Working Group/Flagship/genetic laboratory", there were more reflective and thoughtful answers that shed light on much of the hidden work that is done to embrace genomics. The response of Participant 54, the clinical lead of one of the Flagship projects, illustrates this (see Box 17.1). Rather than just saying, "I lead the team to produce the evidence base for genomic diagnostics in my specialty", they spoke about *liaising, encouraging, supporting* and *explaining* the project. This behind-the-scenes work is clearly an important aspect of their role and one which they have reflected upon, but which is unlikely to be part of their official job description as a Flagship leader.

Box 17.1   First text extract, Participant 54

"I oversee [one of the] Flagships. I work a lot behind the scenes on implementation challenges (lab liaison for example), supporting the project officer
and genetic counsellor, encouraging the flagship clinicians, and explaining
the project to those outside Australian Genomics, who have a tendency to
be sceptical about the value or workability of the project."

The response of Participant 70 reflected their role as a pioneer of sequencing
and genomic diagnostics in Australia (see Box 17.2). This historical perspective
is often lacking, and younger clinicians and scientists as well as non-genetic specialists may be unaware of the prior work that formed the context for their current endeavours. Moreover, translational research networks such as Australian
Genomics often mark their timeline from the date funding was granted with little
reference to antecedents on which they were built. Sharing both these perspectives with the broader membership of Australian Genomics adds richness and perspective to a collective endeavour that relies on collaborative relationships.

Box 17.2   Second text extract, Participant 70

"The [specialist genetic] Unit, because of me and the team in the lab, along
with [biomedical facility], was one of the first diagnostic laboratories in Australia to embrace genomic diagnostics. We established a genomic diagnostic service for [disorders] which has become the standard national referral
pathway for this."

The Capability, Opportunity, and Motivation framework for Behaviour
(COM.B) (Michie, Van Stralen, and West 2011) provides a useful, easy-to-
comprehend structure for communicating findings and co-designing solutions
with study participants to problems that are revealed in interview data. Data are
initially analyzed for barriers and enablers to implementation, before being analyzed to ascertain if each barrier or enabler is either a result of the participants'
capability, opportunities available to them in the workplace or their motivation.
Using the COM.B framework to analyze interview data in this study, we identified
a range of themes about the determinants of implementation of clinical genomics.
Falling within the Motivation domain, participants identified the importance of
customizing information about clinical genomics, so that it is relevant for different
audiences such as patients, hospital executives, policy makers and fellow clinicians. From initial clinician and patient discussions, ongoing clinician and scientist

interactions and dialogues about the organization, the need to have a common understanding of genetics and genomics was highlighted. This included greater community understanding and 'genetic literacy', and the need for scientists and clinicians to speak the same language. From the Opportunity domain, the role of strategic and clinical leadership was highlighted as essential to facilitate the introduction of clinical genomics as a new and potentially disruptive clinical practice:

> Leadership or [a] champion [facilitates implementation] . . . especially in some areas [where] they're already fairly advanced in using or integrating genomics into their practice. Whereas others, particularly the more service areas, you know, they probably don't understand, and they haven't had a call for it – it's not quite that – that sort of, momentum hasn't really got to them yet.
>
> [Interviewee 5, medical specialist]

Finally, within the Capability domain, the value of informal learning was raised, for example:

> There's no substitute for actually doing the work. Getting your hands dirty, so up until that point [availability of genomic testing], you know, all we could do was send samples to other parts of the world and wait for results to come back.
>
> [Interviewee 3, clinical specialist]

'Hands-on' learning and informal discussion provided an environment where clinicians new to genomics could take in the complexity of the process required to use genomics in practice.

Figures 17.2 and 17.3 show two process maps generated for the project from two different KidGen clinics in different states. Despite the common vision of KidGen,

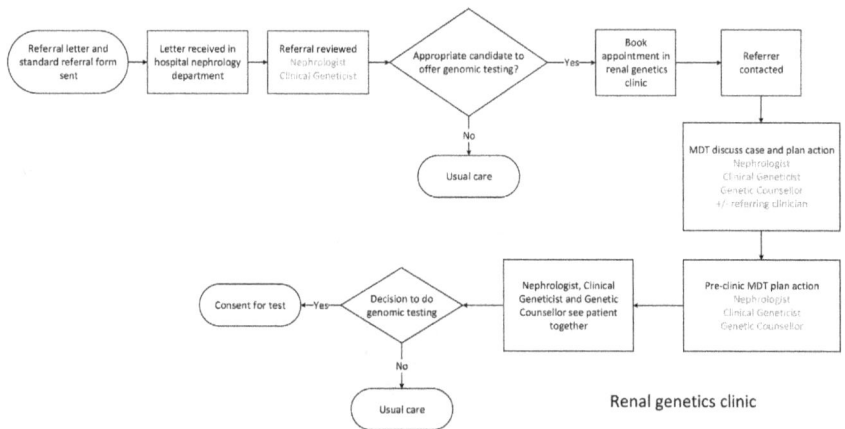

Figure 17.2 Process map of the renal genetics clinic at Site A from receipt of referral to consent for genomic sequencing.

Source: Authors' own work.

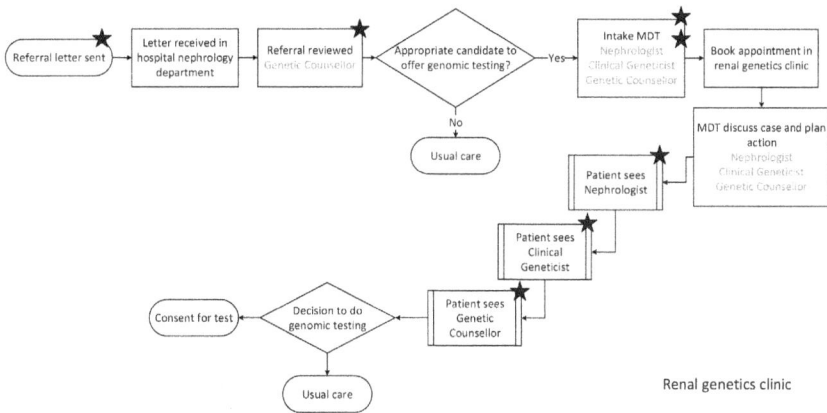

Figure 17.3 Process map of the renal genetics clinic at Site B from receipt of referral to consent for genomic sequencing.

Source: Authors' own work. Stars (★) indicate differences from Site A.

and an expectation that processes would be the same in order to achieve common goals, a range of differences was found in the two process maps in terms of staff numbers in each clinic, types of roles, configuration of teams and the timing of various activities essential for genomic testing. For example, Site A and Site B (Figures 17.2 and 17.3) show differences in the timing of multidisciplinary team meetings, in how the process of genetic variant interpretation was managed, and in how the patient clinics were organized.

Discussion

The three methods – free text survey responses, semi-structured interviews and process mapping – provide a classic triangulation of qualitative data in genomics investigations, securing different standpoints on the implementation of genomics into clinical practice. The free text survey responses offered a personal perspective, the interviews provided both an individual view and also drew out organizational influences, and the process maps aided understanding of organizational operationalization of genomics in the hospital clinic setting.

Overarchingly, we found:

- No singular route, which can be agreed on by all, about how to secure the application of genomics into practice.
- Many implementation challenges are either hidden or not well understood.
- The significance of first-hand experience, presented through rich, qualifying statements, of being involved with genomic research, technology and medicine.

Identified gaps in getting genomics into practice	Links	Themes for our research
1) translation from laboratory procedure to clinical practice		a) the need for packaging information to ensure it is accessible for different audiences
		b) the importance of clinical leadership
2) transition from a clinical research practice to standard clinical care		c) the impact of past endeavours in shaping the current context

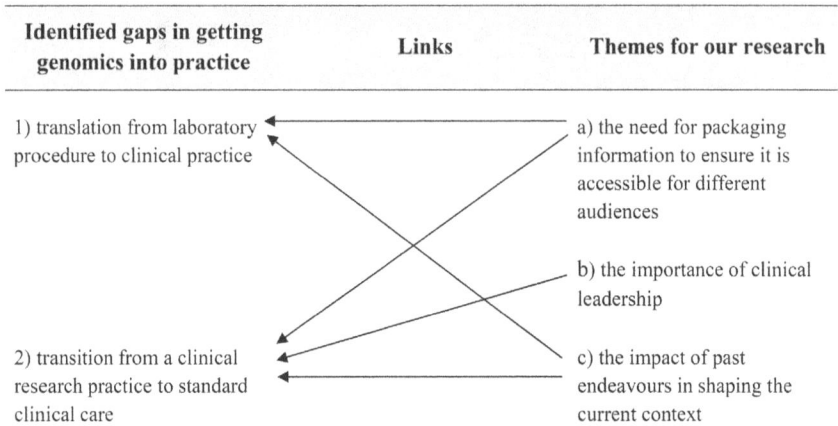

Figure 17.4 Linking themes from the data to known translation gaps.
Source: Authors' own work.

In practice, genomic implementation must build on the foundations laid by previous, often ground-breaking services and earlier thinking about adoption, taking as a departure point existing infrastructure and staff resources. We found three recurring themes across the different research approaches: a) the need to customize the presentation of information to ensure it is accessible for different audiences, b) the importance of clinical leadership in making progress, and c) the impact of past and present contextual factors on how genomic services evolve. These three themes feed directly into the frontline genomic implementation gaps we discerned from this work (Figure 17.4).

The process mapping work showed that, even with an explicit shared goal (Mallett et al. 2016) (getting genomics into the clinic and routine practice) and some standardization within a research project context, clinical processes varied markedly. The survey elicited stories placing current genomic work in the context of 30 years of genetic services and molecular diagnostics and gave insights into important behind-the-scenes work. The interviews gave more scope for an in-depth analysis of how some early adopters of genomic practice viewed the issues.

Implications for practice and theory

Each of the themes (Figure 17.4) identified can be fostered as potential solutions. Theme a) *the need to present information for different audiences* is imperative to see the move of genomics from the laboratory and then out of the research environment into real world contexts (Manolio et al. 2013). This was made clear from the interviews with a range of stakeholders. While commissioners of services, clinicians and consumers believe genomics is largely the preserve of researchers it will likely remain 'stuck', unable to make the move into routine clinical practice (Khoury et al. 2007). Implementation of clinical genomics will require much broader input from clinicians, service providers and the community. The survey response from the Flagship leaders also gave an insight into the need to explain the project to people outside Australian Genomics, who feel implementation will flow naturally and effortlessly on from research based projects. This supports the view that we need to take a tailored approach to information giving and information sharing.

Theme b) *clinical leadership* highlights the need to influence the move from technical research into mainstream clinical care. Interviews with clinicians and service level influencers in particular, made it clear that the role of clinicians, to translate laboratory findings into clinically meaningful actions, is an essential first step. This is closely followed by championing the use of genomics, not only with fellow clinicians but at a hospital board level too. Clinical leadership was identified as key to fostering the development of genomics in clinical practice but also to support the growth of new emerging specialist clinicians who are pushing the boundaries of what is known and what can be done both in the clinic and with the laboratory scientists. Traversing the sociotechnical space that genomics represents is challenging in many respects, and clinicians engaged in this field will, over time, benefit from the support of local clinical leaders to fulfil the promise of genomics.

Theme c) *the impact of past endeavours in shaping the current context* encouraged personal reflections on one's role in achieving the aims of Australian Genomics and illuminated two potential solutions. The Flagship leader who emphasized their hidden work in making the Flagship-initiated processes successful in the first instance, and sustainable beyond the research funding, makes an important point (namely that many processes are social and informal). This should be discussed and encouraged among clinical leaders. Second, the narratives around the first endeavours in genomic work could be disseminated to help early adopters of genomics understand the nature and reasons behind 'the way things are'. Constraining factors such as seemingly-at-odds funding arrangements, inefficient processes or partners that appear mismatched, are better understood when their history is known. For example, understanding that an inefficient process is the legacy of a now redundant test, frees clinicians to remodel the workflow into a new, more efficient one. An appreciation of the history of progress towards implementation of genomics can also aid restructuring processes and understanding crucial interdependencies that make a system work.

Conclusion

The translation of genomic medicine into clinical practice is complex (Chambers, Feerp, and Khoury 2016), demanding a multifaceted approach to implementation. The three methods underpinning implementation science approaches outlined in this chapter show the depth of data that can be uncovered with qualitative research methods. It is on the basis of this qualitative information that progress towards routinizing genomics into practice can be made.

References

Australian Genomic Health Alliance. 2018. "Australian genomic health alliance." Accessed July 2018. www.australiangenomics.org.au/.

Biesecker, LG, and RC Green. 2014. "Diagnostic clinical genome and exome sequencing." *New England Journal of Medicine* 370 (25):2418–2425.

Chalmers, I, and P Glasziou. 2009. "Avoidable waste in the production and reporting of research evidence." *The Lancet* 374 (9683):86–89.

Chambers, DA, W Feerp, and M Khoury. 2016. "Convergence of implementation science, precision medicine, and the learning health care system: A new model for biomedical research." *JAMA* 315 (18):1941–1942.

Khoury, M, M Gwinn, P Yoon, N Dowling, C Moore, and L Bradley. 2007. "The continuum of translation research in genomic medicine: How can we accelerate the appropriate integration of human genome discoveries into health care and disease prevention?" *Genetics in Medicine* 9 (10):665–674.

Korf, B. 2002. "Genetics in medical practice." *Genetics in Medicine* 4 (S6):10s–14s.

Long, JC, C Pomare, S Best, T Boughtwood, K North, LA Ellis, . . . J Braithwaite. 2019. "Building a learning community of Australian clinical genomics: A social network study of the Australian genomic health alliance." *BMC Medicine* 17 (44).

Mallett, A, L Fowles, J McGaughran, H Healy, and C Patel. 2016. "A multidisciplinary renal genetics clinic improves patient diagnosis." *Medical Journal of Australia* 204:57–59.

Manolio, TC, RL Chisholm, B Ozenberger, D Roden, M Williams, R Wilson, D Bick, . . . G Ginsburg. 2013. "Implementing genomic medicine in the clinic: The future is here." *Genetics in Medicine* 15 (4):253–267.

Michie, S, MM Van Stralen, and R West. 2011. "The behaviour change wheel: A new method for characterising and designing behaviour change interventions." *Implementation Science* 6 (1):42.

Stark, Z, D Schofield, K Alam, W Wilson, N Mupfeki, I Macciocca, . . . C Gaff. 2017. "Prospective comparison of the cost-effectiveness of clinical whole-exome sequencing with that of usual care overwhelmingly supports early use and reimbursement." *Genetics in Medicine* 19 (8):867–874.

Taylor, N, S Best, M Martyn, JC Long, KN North, J Braithwaite, and C Gaff. 2019. "A transformative translational change programme to introduce genomics into healthcare: A complexity and implementation science study protocol." *BMJ Open* 9 (3):e024681.

Walsh, M, M Bell Katrina, B Chong, E Creed, R Brett Gemma, K Pope, . . . M Ryan Monique. 2017. "Diagnostic and cost utility of whole exome sequencing in peripheral neuropathy." *Annals of Clinical and Translational Neurology* 4 (5):318–325.

Wolf, SM, LM Amendola, JS Berg, WK Chung, EW Clayton, RC Green, . . . BA Koenig. 2018. "Navigating the research – clinical interface in genomic medicine: Analysis from the CSER consortium." *Genetics in Medicine* 20 (5):545.

18 Much more than old wine in new bottles

Soft Systems Methodology (SSM) for healthcare improvement

Hanna Augustsson, Kate Churruca and Jeffrey Braithwaite

Introduction

Change is the reality of everyday life in healthcare, not least because of accelerating medical, technological and social advances, and shifting models of care. As a consequence, health systems must continuously assess and update the ways in which they operate as well as the methods of change. However, implementation and improvement efforts in healthcare have proven to be challenging (Brownson, Colditz, and Proctor 2018; Grimshaw et al. 2012; Greenhalgh et al. 2004; Grol and Grimshaw 2003; Rapport et al. 2018).

Addressing the task of improvement and evaluation can be understood in light of the sheer complexity of healthcare (Plsek and Greenhalgh 2001; Braithwaite 2018). Healthcare organizations and systems comprise a range of interdependent components – artefacts, buildings, equipment, processes, individuals and groups – which interact in ways that are impossible to fully predict, and that flex and adapt over time (Braithwaite et al. 2018). The intense interconnectedness and yet paradoxical divisions and silos separating agents across their differing contexts implies that sometimes a change in one part of the system, even a seemingly small one, can perturb other parts of the system (known as the butterfly effect (Lorenz 1993)) whereas an attempt at universal transformation (e.g., a major structural change) can have minimal impact (Plsek and Greenhalgh 2001). Clearly, the interdependent and dynamic nature of healthcare means that the context will differ across organizations, between different parts of an organization as well as over different hierarchies and heterarchies within organizations. All of this implies that even in principle, let alone in practice, there is no one-size-fits-all solution when it comes to implementing improvements in healthcare. Furthermore, evaluation of progress when change is enabled becomes a problem not just because of this complexity, but because evaluators are trying to assess an unpredictable, moving target, with behaviours that are emergent rather than stable or forecastable.

Despite this, positivist and reductionist methods such as Randomized Controlled Trials (RCTs) and top-down interventions have often been considered the gold standard when it comes to demonstrating change in care systems. Yet, RCTs and other meticulous research designs, and above-down systems-level interventions, implicitly assume control of the context. This fails to recognize context as an inevitable element in any change, both influencing it and being influenced by it (Kessler and Glasgow 2011; May, Johnson, and Finch 2016; Greenhalgh and Papoutsi 2018; Cohn et al. 2013). In fact, linear models have been tried many times and, even when they are successful, effect sizes are modest (Grimshaw et al. 2012). From this it follows that, in searching for solutions, we must become more attuned to exploring multifaceted and context-dependent strategies for improvement.

One approach for factoring in, rather than ignoring, the complexity of context is Soft Systems Methodology (SSM), first pioneered by Checkland and colleagues in the 1970s and 1980s (Checkland 1981; Checkland and Poulter 2006) and discussed with application to healthcare by Hindle and Braithwaite almost two decades ago (Braithwaite et al. 2002; Hindle and Braithwaite 2002). SSM has demonstrated efficacy as a social, qualitative method for tackling problems that are incredibly hard to solve, or even impossible to solve fully ('wicked problems') (Rittel and Webber 1973) in non-health settings (Ackermann 2012; Mingers and White 2010; Rosenhead 1996), but has been only sporadically and typically inconsistently applied in healthcare (Augustsson, Churruca, and Braithwaite Forthcoming; Hindle and Braithwaite 2002).

SSM falls into the category of action research (Greenwood and Levin 2007; Meyer 2000), directly involving a group of key stakeholders who essentially need to begin with a problem situation, which then stimulates their improvement efforts. This is in contrast, for example, to the change process being driven by researchers or senior managers. SSM is designed to acknowledge the complexities of the real world rather than settling for simplified or idealized solutions that all-too-often do not work in practice.

In this chapter we explore the role and future potential of SSM to facilitate change in healthcare, beginning with a description of the methodology. We then provide illustrative health-related examples of how SSM has been used in healthcare. We then extract the main principles from our analysis of SSM that can support, at least in theory, more responsive, sustainable change. SSM comes with its own technical language for which we provide definitions, based on Checkland's original writings (Box 18.1), aspects of which will be clarified in more detail in the following sections where we examine SSM more fully.

Box 18.1 Description of key terms and tools used in SSM

Rich picture – Exploration of the problematical situation and description of it by making drawings of the situation, including the various stakeholders' roles, structures and processes as well as the relationships between these.

Purposeful activity – Any activity that is goal-directed and useful; defined by a transformation process, i.e. an input being transformed to an output, within the scope of a worldview (see 'CATWOE').

Purposeful activity model (PAM) – A conceptual model, based on one declared worldview, for one or more aspects of the problematical situation outlining a set of purposeful activities relevant to the situation. The model is a set of linked activities that together makes up a purposeful whole.

Root definition – A statement describing the PAM to be modelled.

CATWOE – A 'reminder' to consider the following information about the situation and the PAM:

- **C**ustomers – The beneficiaries or victims affected by the problematical situation and the improvement intervention.
- **A**ctors – The individuals involved in performing the improvement.
- **T**ransformation – The change process, i.e. an input being transformed to an output.
- **W**orldview – Underlying assumptions that make the improvement intervention worthwhile and important (also known as weltanschauung in SSM).
- **O**wners – The actors that are responsible for the improvement intervention and who decide whether it will be implemented or not.
- **E**nvironmental constraints and enablers – The contextual factors that may influence the problematical situation and the improvement intervention.

The PQR formula – A formula useful for defining the root definition. It is applied by answering the questions: what should be done (P), how it should be done (Q) and why it should be done (R).

Five Es – Criteria for assessing the outcomes of the improvement intervention, including:

- **Efficacy** – Does the intervention produce the intended outcomes?
- **Efficiency** – Is the improvement being achieved with minimum use of resources?
- **Effectiveness** – Does the intervention help achieve some higher-level or longer-term aim?
- **Ethicality** – Is the intervention morally correct?
- **Elegance** – Is it an aesthetically pleasing transformation?

Pathways to addressing problems: soft systems methodology explained

SSM is an approach designed for tackling real world, messy, challenging problems. At its heart it is a learning process – one that engages relevant stakeholders in a method of inquiry into a problematic situation with the aim of improving it. The methodology involves four activities:

Activity 1. Finding out about the problematical situation.
Activity 2. Constructing conceptual models called Purposeful Activity Models (PAMs).
Activity 3. Comparing the conceptual models to the 'real world'.
Activity 4. Taking action to improve (Checkland and Poulter 2006).

These activities are supported by several SSM tools. The four activities and the supporting tools need a brief introduction to those not well versed in SSM's methods, as defined in Box 18.1. For a more comprehensive description of the complete methodology see for instance Checkland and Poulter (2006).

Activity 1. *Finding out about the problematical situation*

The first activity, which we have come to think about as '*a picture tells a thousand words*', is concerned with understanding the challenge selected for SSM action, and the circumstances in which the problem may have arisen. It is important to include stakeholders with different views about the situation in order to capture varying perspectives and secure as comprehensive a picture of the situation as possible. Information about the situation is often collected through interviews or focus groups but other methods such as observations, document analysis and surveys can also be used. The exploration involves analysis of: 1) the proposed intervention itself, including the actors involved; 2) the socio-cultural context including roles, norms and values; and 3) existing power structures. The supporting tool for this activity is the *rich picture* – an illustration of the problem and its context, describing the situation in drawings or diagrams, helping to elucidate the links between different factors, actors, processes and structures.

Activity 2. *Constructing PAMs*

In the second activity, conceptual models known as Purposeful Activity Models (PAMs) are constructed. A PAM is not a description of how the situation is *per se* but instead *outlines a system of relevant purposeful activities for the situation, based on a single worldview*. In order to construct the PAM, a statement describing the activity system to be modelled is needed. This statement in SSM language is a *root definition*. Formulation of root definitions can be facilitated by using the *PQR formula* which poses the questions: what should be done (P), how should it be done (Q), and why should it be done (R)? Another supporting tool is the *CATWOE* mnemonic which helps to identify relevant Customers, Actors, Transformations, Worldviews, Owners and Environmental constraints involved in the situation (Box 18.1). This information can be used to supplement the root definition and make sure that all relevant information is included in the analysis and modelling. The root definition, and in particular the transformation process, are important in order to construct the model since a PAM is basically a description of the purposeful activities needed to perform a transformation – the name given by SSM to the change proposed. Performance measures, which are criteria used to define and monitor the performance of the PAM, are also defined in this activity. This is often referred to as the *three Es* – Efficacy, Efficiency and Effectiveness. This set of core criteria can be extended by adding Elegance and Ethicality, bringing them to *five Es* (Checkland 2000).

Activity 3. Comparing the conceptual model to the 'real world'

In the third SSM activity, which we think of as *"bridging the world-as-imagined so it is in line with the world-as-done"* (Braithwaite, Wears, and Hollnagel 2016), the PAMs are compared with how the 'real world' situation is, and feasible and desirable changes are discussed. Hence, a PAM developed in the previous step does not represent a perfect solution that should be implemented unquestioningly but can be used to stimulate debate about what changes are needed and desirable as well as feasible to implement. Another aim of this activity is to encourage settlement between conflicting views which will enable improvement actions to be taken. This recognizes the well-worn point that there are always conflicting views in healthcare – doctors, nurses and allied health practitioners differ in their perspectives from each other, for example, and managers, policymakers and patients also have distinguishable vantage points on issues facing them.

Activity 4. Taking action to improve

In the fourth activity, which we call the '*change-in-context, realized*', the changes that have been identified as desirable and feasible are implemented and evaluated. This should be seen as a cyclical rather than linear process including instituting a change, assessing its progress formatively and making refinements or decisions to test another consequential change, and so forth. The same is true for the entire SSM process. Even though we are describing it in a roughly linear manner here, it is messier than this description implies; the SSM process is oftentimes iterative, sometimes circular and occasionally cascading, and going back and forth between the activities is normal.

How SSM has been applied in healthcare

We turn to an overview of a selection of studies that have used SSM for improvements in different ways and give illustrative examples of how SSM has been mobilized. Studies articulating SSM show that the methodology has been very broadly, and inconsistently, applied in the healthcare context. The range of foci for SSM solutions has been wide, including policy settings (Vandenbroeck et al. 2014; Kalim, Carson, and Cramp 2006), hospitals (Mukotekwa and Carson 2007; Holm, Dahl, and Barra 2013; Emes et al. 2017), aged care (Reed et al. 2007), mental health (Gibb et al. 2002; Pentland et al. 2014), primary care (Darzentas and Spyrou 1993) and community care (O'Meara 2003; Connell et al. 1998). In the hands of its proponents SSM has often been seen as flexible, and suitable for many different kinds of problems. For instance, Emes et al. (2017) harnessed SSM to understand tensions in the discharge process at a hospital. This led to suggestions for how the discharge process could be improved, creating strategies for implementation. Vandenbroeck et al. (2014) had recourse to SSM in setting up a participatory process to lay down solutions to future Belgian child and adolescent mental health care services which resulted in multiple strategic recommendations being put forward. SSM has also been applied in combination with other methods. For instance, Holm, Dahl, and Barra (2013) used SSM in combination with Discrete Event Simulation to develop a decision aid for how to meet surgical demands in a hospital surgery unit. Several improvement actions that would directly and indirectly impact the surgical activity were suggested and subsequently implemented. Table 18.1 outlines selected additional examples of how SSM has been applied in healthcare.

SSM does not prescribe what data collection methods should be applied. However, as illustrated in Table 18.1, interviews or focus groups or discussion groups have often been used to gain an understanding about the problem situation and to inform the construction of PAMs.

Overarchingly, SSM emphasizes the importance of securing the perspectives from different stakeholders involved in or affected by the situation, which is reflected by the, mainly, large number of stakeholder groups consulted in the process. Table 18.1 also highlights the divergent use of different SSM features and tools. While some studies have applied the whole SSM process, including the featured tools, others have chosen only parts of the method or specific tools of the methodology.

All-in-all, SSM has often been used as a problem structuring methodology, aiming to analyze a problem situation to more fully understand it before deciding on what actions are needed to improve it. Often this problem-structuring approach has resulted in a set of changes or recommendations being proposed. However, it is rarer that the studies describe the implementation of the proposed changes or evaluate their outcomes. Because of this, it is our assessment that SSM has not yet been fully exploited in healthcare, nor have its potential advantages been fully evaluated.

Applying SSM principles to support responsive, sustainable or transformative change

Although, as we have seen, SSM has been articulated in a variety of ways, e.g. using different components of the methodology or via a select use of its tools drawn from the larger toolkit, there are some identifiable core components and features of the methodology and its application that we believe are especially useful for enacting change in healthcare.

Table 18.1 Exemplars of SSM in use

Type of problem situation	Setting	Data collection and no. of stakeholder groups consulted	Featured SSM tools	Solution	Outcome
Policy-implementation of diabetes National Service Framework (NSF) (Kalim, Carson, and Cramp 2006).	National Health Services (NHS), United Kingdom.	Interviews. Two stakeholder groups.	Rich picture, CATWOE,[1] root definition, PAM,[2] comparison of PAM and the real world situation.	Issues relating to human communication, information provision and resource allocation were identified and desirable and feasible changes to achieve a more effective NSF implementation were proposed.	N/K
Knowledge management in mental health (Pentland et al. 2014).	Specialist mental health service, United Kingdom.	Focus groups interviews. Eight stakeholder groups.	Rich picture, root definition, PQR,[3] PAM.	Four key changes for how to improve the knowledge management system were proposed.	Substantial changes were made to the ways in which the teams acquired, stored and shared information about research knowledge.
Development of context-appropriate informatics tools (Unertl et al. 2009).	Ambulatory care, United States of America.	Interviews, observations. Seven stakeholder groups.	Rich picture.	A framework of ten guidelines for the design and implementation of health information technology solutions for chronic disease care were developed.	N/K
Continuity of care (Price and Lau 2013).	Palliative care in two communities, Canada.	Interviews, discussion groups. Nine stakeholder groups.	Rich picture, PAM.	An extended circle of care model of continuity of care which can be used by health planners as they consider changes to policy and practice was developed.	N/K
Complex care pathway (Crowe et al. 2017).	Multiple sectors, United Kingdom.	Interviews, systematic review, online discussion forum, national CHD[4] and paediatric intensive care audit datasets. 12 stakeholder groups.	Rich picture, CATWOE, Root definition, PAM.	Evidence-informed recommendations for service improvement for congenital heart disease services were developed.	A coherent set of targeted recommendations for service improvement fed into national decisions about service provision and commissioning.

1 CATWOE is a mnemonic which helps to identify relevant Customers, Actors, Transformations, Worldviews, Owners and Environmental constraints.
2 PAM: Purposeful Activity Models.
3 PQR refers to the PQR formula which poses the questions: what should be done (P), how should it be done (Q), and why should it be done (R)?
4 CHD: Congenital Heart Disease.

Participation

Participatory approaches are emphasized as key to address the challenge of implementation and improvements in healthcare (Churruca et al. 2019). The participatory nature of SSM, with its propensity for involvement of various stakeholders with contextual knowledge, can facilitate a multifaceted and comprehensive understanding of the situation in which the problem exists as well as stimulating adaptations of improvements to fit the local context. Participation can also help to create buy-in from the stakeholders striving to implement the change by raising awareness of the need for change (Armenakis, Harris, and Mossholder 1993). Also, individuals are more likely to support a change effort if they have been involved in forming the solution (Weiner 2009). Moreover, the potential impact of participation does not stop at the particular change effort. By being involved in the SSM process stakeholders are provided with indirect training and tools that can be used beyond the particular problem situation which may help to build capacity for future change efforts (Leeman et al. 2015).

Whole systems perspective

In SSM, a whole problem situation is considered, including the various interlinkages between actors, groups, structures and processes. This is in contrast to trying to control context and isolate interventions in order to assess their effectiveness. The whole systems perspective inevitably makes change management more challenging. Nevertheless, it provides a more comprehensive picture of the situation and potential barriers and facilitators that may impact on a change effort – which sets up better preparedness for the challenges of change management in real world contexts. This knowledge can be used to adapt improvement actions, or context, accordingly (Baker et al. 2015). Another advantage of the whole systems approach is that it helps to detect unintended consequences of a change which may otherwise have been missed by other, more narrow-cast or superficial change initiatives (Braithwaite et al. 2017).

Approaching change in an iterative manner

Regardless of any efforts made to adapt an improvement to the local context and obviate barriers for its implementation, it is impossible to fully predict how a change will unfold in a complex healthcare setting. SSM addresses this by approaching change as an iterative learning process proceeding from finding out about the problematical situation to taking action to improve it and then repeating this cycle. In SSM, this learning process is continuously monitored to assess progress and potential problems. The feedback generated can be used to make quick and timely refinements and adaptations of the improvement effort, making it more likely to achieve sustainable outcomes (Chambers, Glasgow, and Stange 2013).

Conclusion

SSM poses an alternative to more linear ways of enacting and evaluating change in healthcare. The methodology involves several features that have the potential to facilitate change in healthcare including involving stakeholders with unique knowledge about the problem situation and the local context, taking a systems approach and considering change in an iterative manner. Although SSM has been used for a range of problems in healthcare and it heralds much promise in future applications, its full potential is yet to be evaluated and realized. Harnessing SSM could support more far-reaching, transformative change via qualitative means, which is a key goal of SSM and this book.

References

Ackermann, F. 2012. "Problem structuring methods 'in the Dock': Arguing the case for Soft OR." *European Journal of Operational Research* 219 (3):652–658.

Armenakis, AA, SG Harris, and KW Mossholder. 1993. "Creating readiness for organizational change." *Human Relations* 46 (6):681–703.

Augustsson, H, K Churruca, and J Braithwaite. Forthcoming. "Change and improvement 50 years in the making: A scoping review of the use of soft systems methodology in healthcare."

Baker, R, J Camosso-Stefinovic, C Gillies, EJ Shaw, F Cheater, S Flottorp, . . . MP Eccles. 2015. "Tailored interventions to address determinants of practice." *Cochrane Database of Systematic Reviews* 4 (April).

Braithwaite, J. 2018. "Changing how we think about healthcare improvement." *BMJ* 361 (k2014).

Braithwaite, J, K Churruca, LA Ellis, J Long, R Clay-Williams, N Damen, . . . K Ludlow. 2017. *Complexity Science in Healthcare – Aspirations, Approaches, Applications and Accomplishments: A White Paper*. Sydney, Australia: Australian Institute of Health Innovation, Macquarie University.

Braithwaite, J, K Churruca, JC Long, LA Ellis, and J Herkes. 2018. "When complexity science meets implementation science: A theoretical and empirical analysis of systems change." *BMC Medicine* 16 (63).

Braithwaite, J, D Hindle, R Iedema, and JI Westbrook. 2002. "Introducing soft systems methodology plus (SSM+): Why we need it and what it can contribute." *Australian Health Review* 25 (2):191–198.

Braithwaite, J, RL Wears, and E Hollnagel. 2016. *Resilient Health Care: Reconciling Work-as-Imagined and Work-as-Done*. Vol. 3. Boca Raton: CRC Press.

Brownson, RC, GA Colditz, and EK Proctor. 2018. *Dissemination and Implementation Research in Health: Translating Science to Practice*. Vol. 2. New York: Oxford University Press.

Chambers, DA, RE Glasgow, and KC Stange. 2013. "The dynamic sustainability framework: Addressing the paradox of sustainment amid ongoing change." *Implementation Science* 8 (117).

Checkland, P. 1981. *Systems Thinking, Systems Practice*. Chichester: John Wiley & Sons, Ltd.

Checkland, P. 2000. "Soft systems methodology: A 30-year retrospective." *Systems Research and Behavioral Science* 17 (S1):S11–S58.

Checkland, P, and J Poulter. 2006. *Learning for Action: A Short Definitive Account of Soft Systems Methodology and Its Use, for Practitioners, Teachers and Students*. Chichester: John Wiley & Sons, Ltd.

Churruca, K, K Ludlow, N Taylor, JC Long, S Best, and J Braithwaite. 2019. "The time has come: Embedded implementation research for health care improvement." *Journal of Evaluation in Clinical Practice* 25 (3):373–380.

Cohn, S, M Clinch, C Bunn, and P Stronge. 2013. "Entangled complexity: Why complex interventions are just not complicated enough." *Journal of Health Services Research & Policy* 18 (1):40–43.

Connell, NAD, AR Goddard, I Philp, and J Bray. 1998. "Patient-centred performance monitoring systems and multi-agency care provision: A case study using a stakeholder participative approach." *Health Services Management Research* 11 (2):92–102.

Crowe, S, K Brown, J Tregay, J Wray, R Knowles, DA Ridout, . . . M Utley. 2017. "Combining qualitative and quantitative operational research methods to inform quality improvement in pathways that span multiple settings." *BMJ Quality & Safety* 26 (8):641–652.

Darzentas, J, and T Spyrou. 1993. "Information systems for primary health care: The case of the Aegean islands." *European Journal of Information Systems* 2 (2):117–127.

Emes, M, S Smith, S Ward, A Smith, and T Ming. 2017. "Care and flow: Using Soft Systems Methodology to understand tensions in the patient discharge process." *Health Systems* 6 (3):260–278.

Gibb, CE, M Morrow, CL Clarke, G Cook, P Gertig, and V Ramprogus. 2002. "Transdisciplinary working: Evaluating the development of health and social care provision in mental health." *Journal of Mental Health* 11 (3):339–350.

Greenhalgh, T, and C Papoutsi. 2018. "Studying complexity in health services research: Desperately seeking an overdue paradigm shift." *BMC Medicine* 16 (95).

Greenhalgh, T, G Robert, F Macfarlane, P Bate, and O Kyriakidou. 2004. "Diffusion of innovations in service organizations: Systematic review and recommendations." *Milbank Quarterly* 82 (4):581–629.

Greenwood, DJ, and M Levin. 2007. *Introduction to Action Research: Social Research for Social Change*. 2nd ed. Thousand Oaks: Sage.

Grimshaw, JM, MP Eccles, JN Lavis, SJ Hill, and JE Squires. 2012. "Knowledge translation of research findings." *Implementation Science* 7 (50).

Grol, R, and J Grimshaw. 2003. "From best evidence to best practice: Effective implementation of change in patients' care." *The Lancet* 362 (9391):1225–1230.

Hindle, D, and J Braithwaite. 2002. *Soft Systems Methodology Plus (SSM+): A Guide for Australian Health Care Professionals*. Sydney: Centre for Clinical Governance Research, University of New South Wales.

Holm, LB, FA Dahl, and M Barra. 2013. "Towards a multimethodology in health care – synergies between soft systems methodology and discrete event simulation." *Health Systems* 2 (1):11–23.

Kalim, K, E Carson, and D Cramp. 2006. "An illustration of whole systems thinking." *Health Services Management Research* 19 (3):174–185.

Kessler, R, and RE Glasgow. 2011. "A proposal to speed translation of healthcare research into practice: Dramatic change is needed." *American Journal of Preventive Medicine* 40 (6):637–644.

Leeman, J, L Calancie, MA Hartman, CT Escoffery, AK Herrmann, LE Tague, . . . C Samuel-Hodge. 2015. "What strategies are used to build practitioners' capacity to implement community-based interventions and are they effective? A systematic review." *Implementation Science* 10 (80).

Lorenz, E. 1993. *The Essence of Chaos*. Seattle: University of Washington Press.

May, CR, M Johnson, and T Finch. 2016. "Implementation, context and complexity." *Implementation Science* 11 (141).

Meyer, J. 2000. "Using qualitative methods in health related action research." *BMJ* 320:178–181.

Mingers, J, and L White. 2010. "A review of the recent contribution of systems thinking to operational research and management science." *European Journal of Operational Research* 207 (3):1147–1161.

Mukotekwa, C, and E Carson. 2007. "Improving the discharge planning process: A systems study." *Journal of Research in Nursing* 12 (6):667–686.

O'Meara, P. 2003. "Would a prehospital practitioner model improve patient care in rural Australia?" *Emergency Medicine Journal* 20:199–203.

Pentland, D, K Forsyth, D Maciver, M Walsh, R Murray, and L Irvine. 2014. "Enabling integrated knowledge acquisition and management in health care teams." *Knowledge Management Research & Practice* 12 (4):362–374.

Plsek, PE, and T Greenhalgh. 2001. "Complexity science: The challenge of complexity in health care." *BMJ* 323:625–628.

Price, M, and FY Lau. 2013. "Provider connectedness and communication patterns: Extending continuity of care in the context of the circle of care." *BMC Health Services Research* 13 (309).

Rapport, F, R Clay-Williams, K Churruca, P Shih, A Hogden, and J Braithwaite. 2018. "The struggle of translating science into action: Foundational concepts of implementation science." *Journal of Evaluation in Clinical Practice* 24 (1):117–126.

Reed, J, P Inglis, G Cook, C Clarke, and M Cook. 2007. "Specialist nurses for older people: Implications from UK development sites." *Journal of Advanced Nursing* 58 (4):368–376.

Rittel, HW, and MM Webber. 1973. "Dilemmas in a general theory of planning." *Policy Sciences* 4 (2):155–169.

Rosenhead, J. 1996. "What's the problem? An introduction to problem structuring methods." *Interfaces* 26 (6):117–131.

Unertl, KM, MB Weinger, KB Johnson, and NM Lorenzi. 2009. "Describing and modeling workflow and information flow in chronic disease care." *Journal of the American Medical Informatics Association* 16 (6):826–836.

Vandenbroeck, P, R Dechenne, K Becher, M Eyssen, and K Van den Heede. 2014. "Recommendations for the organization of mental health services for children and adolescents in Belgium: Use of the soft systems methodology." *Health Policy* 114 (2–3):263–268.

Weiner, BJ. 2009. "A theory of organizational readiness for change." *Implementation Science* 4 (67).

19 Conclusion

On progress, directions and signposts to a transformed healthcare system

Jeffrey Braithwaite and Frances Rapport

Prologue

In Phillip Pullman's fantasy masterpiece, the trilogy *His Dark Materials* (Pullman 2011), the heroine, pre-teen Lyra Belacqua takes possession of an Alethiometer – an imaginary device resembling a cross between a compass and a pocket watch. Laden with symbols, it tells the truth in response to any question asked by a trained or intuitively skilled operator by the hands moving to point to the symbols. Armed with this information, the enquirer can then decide what to do next. With answers to her queries, Lyra can make her way in the world, solving problems along the way in her journey of discovery.

That is as good an analogy as any for the compass that is this book. It offers evidence-based and theoretically-grounded pointers to the future for those who are interested in transforming healthcare. It helps by uncovering what is happening now in different health systems and parts of health systems. The researchers-explorers of this volume provide detailed and rich information across the pages of their chapters on which those in the system can base their improvement efforts.

It is our task in this chapter to bring all that Alethiometer-like information in the book into focus and together, acting as we believe it does, as a series of signposts for future reform efforts. We do not have the 36 symbols of an Alethiometer, but 19 chapters (including this one) which serve as our gateway into the system we wish to understand and enhance.

Reading the Alethiometer of transformation

After the descriptive and analytic work is over, qualitative researchers often move on to present their work through articles, conference proceedings, books and book chapters, invariably incorporating theories or drawing on empirical methods, or both, to tell a story through their accounts. The present chapters in this book are no exception, providing a 'window of understanding' through the accumulation of narrative trajectories, and the features, characteristics and context of the topic each author or author group chooses to tackle.

As we traverse the chapters, we can discern across the pages plenty of wisdom and scholarship. Each author or author group chose problems in which they had expertise and rendered a well-grounded description of the issues they faced in addressing these issues. They adduced, analysed or synthesised research, or applied, explained or mobilised theories, or both, to make sense of their particular topic. Each chapter, Alethiometer-like, reveals multiple truths, and signals how care works or doesn't work, or how it might work better, in the particular domain of choice. The chapters come together to provide a composite picture of health-care – offering a 'direction-finder' to transformed care in the future.

When we asked our authors to contribute, we didn't discuss Alethiometers, the other authors or the topics in the rest of the book. We simply asked them to provide a chapter of qualitative research in their domain of expertise. Nor did we say, "no numbers allowed", although it is true to say there are not many numbers across the pages of the book. What we did emphasise was our interest in real world descriptions, bolstered where authors thought it necessary by pictures and graph-ics by which they could portray their particular interest in their healthcare topic of choice. By asking them to focus on transforming healthcare, we did not neces-sarily mean "big picture, systems-wide reform, restructuring or reorganisation", although that is often what is meant by 'transformation'. In point of fact, there are not many chapters with a whole system focus. Health systems can be transformed by endeavours at macro, meso and micro levels, and across the aged, community, rehabilitation, acute, general practice or mental health sectors, or indeed, at sub-sector level too. Localised, or modest improvements can be a harbinger of larger change, if scaled. That is what we see here.

Ways and means of transforming healthcare

Against this backdrop of understanding what the chapter authors did, and how they responded to our request for involvement, we want to turn to what we have taken away to act as an Alethiometer-inspired wayfinder for our readers. Although a summary table runs the risk of unduly simplifying the rich narratives that the individual chapters provide, we have opted to provide this by way of document-ing in one place the key lessons, transformational implications, provenance of authors, types of studies and sites of research, and empirical and theoretical foci as we read and distilled them (Table 19.1). Following that, we have made word clouds of each chapter, each of the three parts (Ideas, Systems and Solutions) and the whole book as a way of providing at-a-glance insights into the essence of the volume and its parts (Figures 19.1–19.23, created using Word Art 2019).

Lessons and signposts: toward a transformed system

This high-level excursion through the pages of the book via two different meth-ods, expert synthesis and auto-generated word cloud generation, encapsuled in Table 19.1 and the word clouds, reveals how the chapter authors have drawn many lessons from their qualitative research and the propensities, possibilities and promises it brings for improving care. They have teased out their topics and put

Table 19.1 Overview of chapters

1 Introduction: First Things First	
Key lessons	Makes the case for the book – showing how interdisciplinary researchers furnished varied perspectives, illuminating how to transform healthcare by leveraging qualitative methods.
	Perspectives include how patients can influence care; ways to enhance patients' journeys through the system; the limits and constraints on delivery systems on how to exploit advances and emerging technologies; new frameworks for change management such as complexity science; novel tools or revamped tools, made fit-for-purpose; and glimpses of future care, tools or models such as in situ simulation, huddles, soft systems methodology, genomic medicine, cross boundary teaming and sensemaking.
Transformational implications	There are many levers for transformational change under the three sections of the book, mapped to Ideas, Systems and Solutions.
Country of author, study, research site	United Kingdom, Australia and all the other countries involved – Canada, Brazil, France, United States of America, Japan and Sweden.
Empirical methods and focus	Outline of the structure of the book, and all methods; overall, the focus of the whole volume.
Theoretical approach	Foreshadowing what will happen next, following this introductory chapter.
2 Qualitative Evidence Synthesis and Conceptual Development	
Key lessons	The medicalisation and care of patients needs to be balanced against the interests, perspectives and wishes of patients. For example, they may not take medicines, or in the way prescribed – but this does not necessarily mean they are to be labelled 'non-adherent'; it may be a rational choice.
	Patients' experiences are synthesised in a series of case studies, via meta-analytic techniques such as concept clarification, line of argument analysis and diagrammatic depiction of concepts.
Transformational implications	Raising the voice of the patient to be more prominent, to balance the dominant paradigm of medico-centrism in health and medicine, would go a long way to address epistemic injustice.
Country of author, study, research site	United Kingdom, medication management in multiple settings.
Empirical methods and focus	Qualitative triangulation and conceptual clarification of multiple, person-centred, ethnographic case study accounts of patients' perspectives.
Theoretical approach	Qualitative synthesis; patient-based; sociological orientation.

	3 The Life-Project of Personal Wellbeing: Modern Healthcare and the Individuality of Health
Key lessons	Argues for the importance of the unique individual, recursively enmeshed in the environment in which he or she occupies a distinctive space. These personal life-worlds lead to individuals bringing their own perspectives on health and well-being.
Transformational implications	Humans have the right to their individuality, and medical recognition of that individuality.
Country of author, study, research site	United Kingdom; individuals and their life-projects.
Empirical methods and focus	Analytical philosophical approach.
Theoretical approach	Anthropological; philosophical; human rights.
	4 Socio-narratology and the Clinical Encounter Between Human Beings
Key lessons	People tell stories in healthcare settings: patients, and clinicians. Stories are about people, places and characters. Narratives are broader: schemas that give shape to stories. Socio-narratives involve social texture: the circumstances, communication, behaviours and interactions around which and within which stories inhere. Seven question-openings of stories as narrative care are proposed. These ask: which are the regular companions of a story-teller; what type of narrative is the story relating to; what is the narrative logic of the story; what characters are being mobilised to tell the story; which communities or stakeholders are involved in or represented by the story; how committed are the teller and listener to the story or narrative; and, what conflicts are created by the story?
Transformational implications	Storytelling helps people make their lives intelligible and coherent; narrative care can transform healthcare one story at a time. Socio-narrative can enlarge people's curiosity and support understanding.
Country of author, study, research site	Canada; patients telling their stories in healthcare settings.
Empirical methods and focus	Stories from the field of health and medicine.
Theoretical approach	Narrative healthcare; socio-narratology.

(Continued)

Table 19.1 (Continued)

5 Interrupted Body Projects and the Narrative Reconstruction of Self	
Key lessons	A special case of narrative is when a person sustains a traumatic event such as a spinal cord injury. While the stories chosen to rely on, while not unlimited, can vary, two specific narratives that are chosen after spinal cord injury are examined: restitution and quest. The restitution narrative has a plotline and is illustrated by cases, e.g., *Dan*: healthy yesterday, sick today, healthy again tomorrow. The quest narrative is more present-focused, but with an arc of progressively being redeemed – hope over time, rather than before and after.
Transformational implications	Lives and systems can be changed when people alter their narrative pathways, especially around a traumatic life event.
Country of author, study, research site	United Kingdom; spinal cord injury patients.
Empirical methods and focus	Cases of spinal cord injury.
Theoretical approach	Narratology; sociologically-grounded.

6 The Fourth Research Paradigm: Activating Researchers For Real World Need	
Key lessons	The first three research paradigms were quantitative, qualitative and mixed methods. We are on the brink of a new paradigm, which incorporates data from the previous three with 'mobile methods' – fluid, emergent data now available from multiple sources including discussions between researchers and those researched; and additionally, digitally-enabled data via handheld devices, phones, apps, wearables, blogs and the like. These can collectively provide rich insights and better interpretations of what is going on in patients' and other stakeholders' lives.
Transformational implications	Research can be transformative in this new model and produce fresh insights into patients' well-being, reactions to treatments, behaviours, attitudes and worldviews.
Country of author, study, research site	Australia; methodologists at the cutting edge of healthcare research.
Empirical methods and focus	Meta-empirical.
Theoretical approach	Information theory; new models and concepts of research.

7 Slack Resources in Healthcare Systems: Waste or Resilience?

Key lessons	As a dynamic, complex socio-technical system, healthcare inevitably creates variability in processes, performance and outcomes. There are also slack resources – those that are available in times of need – but which carry a cost. Too much slack equates with waste; too little, and the system can become stretched and brittle. The two case studies presented are of ward staff preparing and administering drugs – one in a publicly funded hospital and the other in a private hospital. Slack has a dual nature – as a source of resilience and of waste.
Transformational implications	Slack can be managed if information about it is made visible, but this would depend for success on a range of features such as how to handle shifting power imbalances, and the impact of different cultures and financial incentives on people's behaviours.
Country of author, study, research site	Brazil; medication safety in acute settings.
Empirical methods and focus	Case study exemplars.
Theoretical approach	Sociotechnical systems theory; conceptual analysis of slack.

8 Using Qualitative Methods to Understand Resilience Expressions in Complex Systems

Key lessons	A patient died during an operation in a major hospital undergoing a new procedure, to implant a valve in the patient. Being new, a number of additional personnel were crowded into the theatre, supporting the operation, and trying to learn from it. The tragic event was attributed, following a root cause analysis, to the overcrowded, noisy theatre, and the surgeon not hearing the radiographer saying where the valve should go. As a consequence, the hospital introduced 'huddles', whereby operating team members talk through what is about to happen, proactively preparing themselves for risks, complexities and eventualities. The result was to enable teams to learn, anticipate, monitor and respond, and strengthen the capacities of teams for resilient performance.
Transformational implications	Hospitals are complex adaptive systems that can learn from successes and failures. In this case, preparedness against future problems was achieved by introducing a tried and tested mechanism, team huddles, to shore up each team's adaptive capacities, and to help members to heedfully inter-relate. Each team in effect was now buffering against future potential breakdowns.
Country of author, study, research site	France, Australia; operating theatre teams responding to a serious adverse event.
Empirical methods and focus	Qualitative case study beginning with a serious adverse event and investigating, through observations, interviews and documentary analysis, the aftermath of the root cause analysis recommendations.
Theoretical approach	Complexity theory; resilience theory; the Resilience Assessment Grid; huddles as a vehicle for change.

(Continued)

Table 19.1 (Continued)

9 Qualitative Assessment to Improve Everyday Activities: Work-As-Imagined and Work-As-Done	
Key lessons	Taking blood from patients for testing purposes in Emergency Departments seems on the face of it (work-as-imagined, WAI) as a relatively simple set of tasks; take the blood, get the pathology results, feed this into the patient's diagnosis and care. The real world of medical work (work-as-done, WAD) is much messier than the idealised world of thinking about it in the executive suite or conceptualising it on the system-designer's desk. Doing a Functional Resonance Analysis Method (FRAM) exercise highlighted this in this study of doctors' venepuncture activities. The FRAM showed hidden functions, multiple triggers and the complexities of real world workflows, 'workarounds' and variability.
Transformational implications	The case study research here helps us to think much more clearly about how work is conducted in situ, and to be much better at designing systems of care, or improving them, matched to the physical actualities and cognitive demands on people doing the work.
Country of author, study, research site	Australia; Emergency Department; doctors collecting blood.
Empirical methods and focus	Case study drawing on ethnographic observations of doctors drawing blood from patients to create a FRAM model.
Theoretical approach	Resilient healthcare; work-as-imagined contrasted with work-as-done.
10 Narrativizing Cancer Patients' Longitudinal Experiences of Care: Qualitative Inquiry into Lived and Online Melanoma Stories	
Key lessons	Two sets of patient narratives provided rich information about the journeys people take and the stories they tell when undergoing care for melanoma. Such patients face tensions, trials and tribulations, and demonstrate resilience in the light of these challenges. Phases of the journey include initiation into the health system; identification of the condition; action, e.g., treatment, or palliation; and adaptation to the 'new normal'. The intensity of patient experience fluctuates depending on the phase, the extent of the problems faced and the capacities of patients to deal with their situations.
Transformational implications	Patients can be empowered by their situation, not just depressed or defeated by it.
Country of author, study, research site	Australia, for ethnographic accounts of seven shadowed melanoma patients; English speaking populations in various countries for 214 online stories of patients accounting for their illness and journey through the systems of care.
Empirical methods and focus	Lived ethnography for seven patients, via interviews and shadowing; online ethnography for content analysis of 214 stories posted online.
Theoretical approach	Paradigmatic-type narrative enquiry; qualitative modelling and synthesis.

11 Look the Other Way: Patient-centred Care Begins with Care for Our Physicians

Key lessons	The focus here is on doctors who face pressures, threats and burdens that put them at risk of burnout. Three narratives written by doctors highlight this situation: the fast-paced, demanding and poorly controlled environments where the patients with their needs just keep coming, leading to psychological, emotional, physical, social and professional challenges.
	The first-person accounts, by an orthopaedic surgeon, a pulmonary and critical care physician, and an emergency doctor, lay bare the intense environments, emanating from patient crises that often create intimidations and unremitting workloads on the doctors involved. Such self-reflection and honest sharing make the writers not victims but connectors with other doctors, and supporters of others facing their own risk of burnout.
Transformational implications	Forewarned is forearmed; doctors are universally under pressure and at risk of stress, depression, suffering, vulnerabilities and burnout. Caring for the carers is critical for effective patient care.
Country of author, study, research site	United States of America, United Kingdom; three published autobiographical texts offering medical practitioners' insights into burnout.
Empirical methods and focus	Narrative analysis, applying a dialogical, performative approach.
Theoretical approach	Applying Frank's five narrative categories (prompts) to the analysis of the texts: resources, circulation, affiliation, identity and stakes (Frank 2012).

12 Resilient Healthcare in Refractory Epilepsy: Illuminating Successful People-centred Care

Key lessons	Those who suffer from refractory epilepsy face seizures that are unresponsive to antiepileptic drugs. Patients are eligible for resective surgery involving the removal of part of the cortex of the brain, an operation that helps two-thirds of patients with refractory epilepsy to be seizure-free.
	Considerable delays are experienced before surgery, but is this treatment gap a positive or negative thing?
	Focusing on barriers to treatment suggests it is negative, but being more thorough, allowing time for clinicians and patients to think through decisions, and focus on psycho-social health and wellbeing might suggest otherwise. This for the most part is the system being adaptive and focused on things going right.
Transformational implications	Many factors need to be considered before such far-reaching surgery as resective surgery is offered, but at the same time this unique operation can transform the lives of long-suffering patients experiencing a severely debilitating disease.
Country of author, study, research site	Australia; two of three centres in New South Wales doing such surgery.
Empirical methods and focus	Qualitative case study involving patients with refractory epilepsy and specialist clinicians attending to their assessment for surgery and care.
Theoretical approach	Work-as-imagined; barriers and facilitators to treatment and care gaps; operating theatres; stakeholder analysis, resilient healthcare.

(Continued)

Table 19.1 (Continued)

13 Sensemaking as a Strategy for Managing Uncertainty: Change and Surprise in Hospital Settings	
Key lessons	Healthcare settings are complex adaptive systems characterised by lack of certainty; unexpected events; nonlinearity; emergence; ongoing, dynamical change; and surprise. Given these features, how can we manage uncertainty?
	Key factors are relationships, communication, shared mental models and sensemaking – co-creating meaning across team members and coming to shared understandings of care, involving care teams and patients collaborating over care implementation and effectively making sense of what is happening on the ground.
	Working therefore on enhancing relationships, building in time for conversation and interaction, and emphasising effective communication all feed into making sense of care parameters and delivery of services.
Transformational implications	Without co-created meaning, collectively making sense of circumstances, and effective relationships and communication, we cannot deliver patient-centred care, nor effectively improve the delivery system.
Country of author, study, research site	United States of America.
Empirical methods and focus	Multiple studies of care teams in acute settings.
Theoretical approach	Complexity theory; conceptualisations of sensemaking; theories of uncertainty, mental models and co-created care.

14 Simulation to Solve Health System Problems	
Key lessons	In situ simulation offers opportunities to practice procedures and techniques that closely replicate everyday clinical work as well as exceptional circumstances and events as close as possible to frontline care activities. This can be contrasted with ordinary training of teams which tends to occur outside the clinical coalface and in mono-disciplinary silos.
	By standardising the cases and situations represented in a simulation, the way individuals and teams react to clinical situations can be a rich source of information and learning. Debriefings of the interactions and behaviours from multiple perspectives can be highly useful for individual and team development.
	In situ simulations, observations of them and debriefings facilitate the gathering of qualitative information which can be highly valuable.
Transformational implications	Input via in situ simulations can contribute to individual and team development, enhance skills and prepare clinicians and teams for real life scenarios and events in a safe environment, risk-free for patients.
Country of author, study, research site	United States of America; simulation; qualitative assessment of in situ simulations; acute care settings with application to other settings.
Empirical methods and focus	Qualitative observational studies of multiple case enquiries into simulations.
Theoretical approach	Simulation theory; sociological understanding of complex clinical team responses to simulated situations.

15 Cross-Boundary Teaming to Establish Resilience Among Isolated 'Silos'

Key lessons	Going beyond mono-disciplinary teams, cross-boundary teaming involves traversing natural silos prevalent throughout healthcare systems. Using a case study of a contrast-enhanced computed tomography arranged for a patient with a history of anaphylaxis to the contrast agent, an analysis of the roles and attitudes of cardiovascular surgeons, ward nurses, the chief nurse, intensivists, patient safety experts, the director of the emergency department, the director of pharmacy and the director of anaesthesia were all involved. A typology of cross-boundary teaming was developed from this case account. Key attributes of an effective cross-boundary teaming involve: establishing the network, setting collaborative goals and sharing them, appreciating the existing silos, arranging and supporting cross-boundary teaming, identifying barriers to teaming through listening to the voices and ensuring psychological safety of participants.
Transformational implications	Teams dealing with complex circumstances can transcend pre-existing work silos and team boundaries and act effectively as a meta-team more effective in dealing with problems, pre-empting problems and problem-solving.
Country of author, study, research site	Japan; study of cross-boundary activities; acute setting.
Empirical methods and focus	Qualitative case study and synthesis of differing roles, perspectives and boundary-crossing behaviours.
Theoretical approach	Medical meta-team work; theories of cross-boundary teams and teaming.

16 "What on Earth Is Going On and What Should I Do Now?" Sensemaking as a Qualitative Process

Key lessons	Assess the role of sensemaking as an explanation of how people in healthcare workplaces make meaning of their work and take collective action based on those meanings. Sensemakers in Weickian terms (Weick 1995) are enacting the environment, constructing and projecting identity and discovering what is going on and what should be done next. Sensemaking can be studied qualitatively, quantitatively or through mixed methods but has predominantly been studied through ethnographic observation. Sensemaking in healthcare occurs under conditions of uncertainty and complexity; it happens typically in fast-paced and time-pressured circumstances; and action taken emerging from sensemaking activities is a basis for organising people, activities and organisations more effectively.
Transformational implications	Sensemaking can be used as a framework for understanding organisational change; to contribute to safer care; to illuminate how clinicians make decisions in situ and as a guiding framework for research in clinical settings.
Country of author, study, research site	Australia; literature and case mentions; mainly acute settings and general practice.
Empirical methods and focus	Weickian sensemaking with applications to healthcare; qualitative, discursive assessments.
Theoretical approach	Sociological; the social psychology of organising.

(Continued)

Table 19.1 (Continued)

17 Deep Inside the Genomics Revolution: On the Frontlines of Care

Key lessons	To create a better health system for patients, the twin problems facing genomics researchers are simply stated: move laboratory findings into clinical practice and make this routine, across-the-board. Qualitative methods are being used to facilitate translation of research findings to the frontlines of care and illuminate new emerging models, and barriers and enablers to care delivery and enhancement. A triangulated data set, taken together, shows that no one-size-fits-all approach will operate in applying genomics in practice; of the challenges such as the role of leadership and the change of culture and mindset needed, many are hidden or poorly understood; and the rich data that arise from a triangulated data set of qualitative findings yield invaluable insights into diffusion of information challenges, and take-up, adoption and spread possibilities.
Transformational implications	The value of multi-perspectival information about large-scale changes is hard to overemphasise; leadership in clinical genomics will be a crucial lever for change; and understanding the past and present of genomics progress can act as a baseline for transformational change in the future.
Country of author, study, research site	Australia; multiple qualitative studies of progress in adoption of Australian genomics; genomics researchers, laboratories and clinics.
Empirical methods and focus	Process mapping of workflows in genetic clinics; attitude surveys of stakeholders looking at perceptions of challenges to adoption; interviews with stakeholders to determine barriers and enablers.
Theoretical approach	Implicit theories of change on the frontlines of care; triangulation of qualitative findings.

18 Much More Than Old Wine in New Bottles: Soft Systems Methodology (SSM) for Healthcare Improvement

Key lessons	While change is a reality in healthcare, implementation and improvement efforts have often been challenging to accomplish, falling short of expectations. Complexity in healthcare systems is a key reason for this. Soft systems methodology (SSM) is a longstanding, action-research approach which factors in systems complexity. Under-utilised in healthcare, it comes with technical language and methodological technologies, but the approach can be synthesised into four staged activities. These are: uncovering the problem, typically by drawing a rich picture of it; building Purposeful Activity Models (PAMs), or ways to proceed including what should be done, by whom, how and why; comparing the real world situation to the PAM, thereby stimulating debate about implementation of solutions, and resolving conflict where possible; and action and implementation, making refinements and learning along the way.
Transformational implications	The uses of SSM are wide, and examples provided include work from studies of the tensions of patient discharges in the UK; establishing participation for child and adolescent mental health services in Belgium; for hospital surgical demands in Norway; and implementing IT for chronic disease care in the USA.

Country of author, study, research site	Sweden, Australia; a multiplicity of studies across policy, aged care, mental health settings, community outreach, ambulatory care and palliative services.
Empirical methods and focus	SSM mechanisms and approaches applied to real world problems via action research techniques.
Theoretical approach	SSM theory; systems theory; complexity theory.
19 Conclusion: On Progress, Directions and Signposts to a Transformed Healthcare System	
Key lessons	Brings the compendium to a close. Synthesises the learnings into one chapter. Gives pointers to the future based on the wayfaring nature of the chapters. Argues that the key to future transformations include leveraging patient power and the positive exploitation of ideas, e.g., resilient healthcare, understanding systems' properties such as slack or complexity, enabling both facilitators and barriers of complex systems to be assessed, mapping patient trajectories, caring for the carers, enabling people through teaming, facilitating peoples' sensemaking, or revolutionising the way care is delivered and enabling greater resilience in healthcare systems and individuals.
Transformational implications	Transformational leverage is available from multiple sources.
Country of author, study, research site	Australia; United Kingdom.
Empirical methods and focus	Content analysis of chapters; future focused.
Theoretical approach	Triangulation of content; narrative-rendering of the key themes of the book.

Source: Authors' own work.

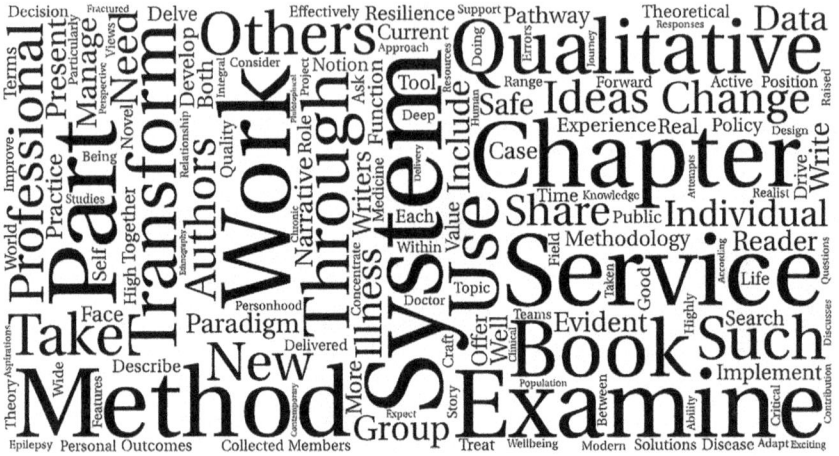

Figure 19.1 Key words relating to Chapter 1.

Source: Authors' own work.

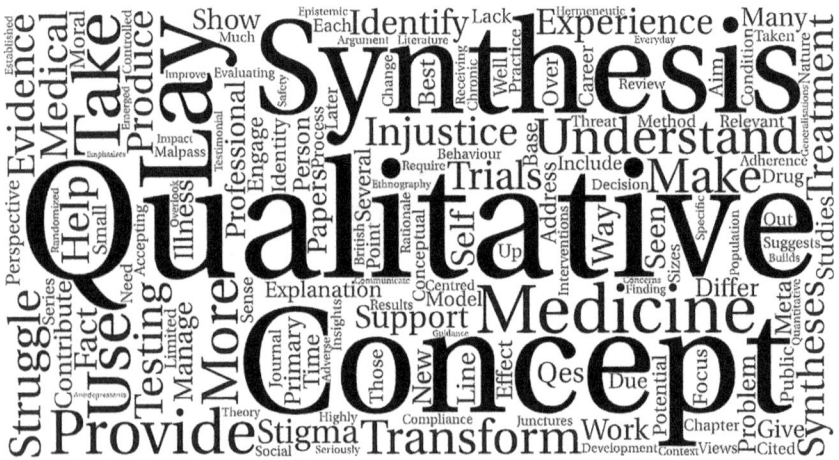

Figure 19.2 Key words relating to Chapter 2.

Source: Author's own work.

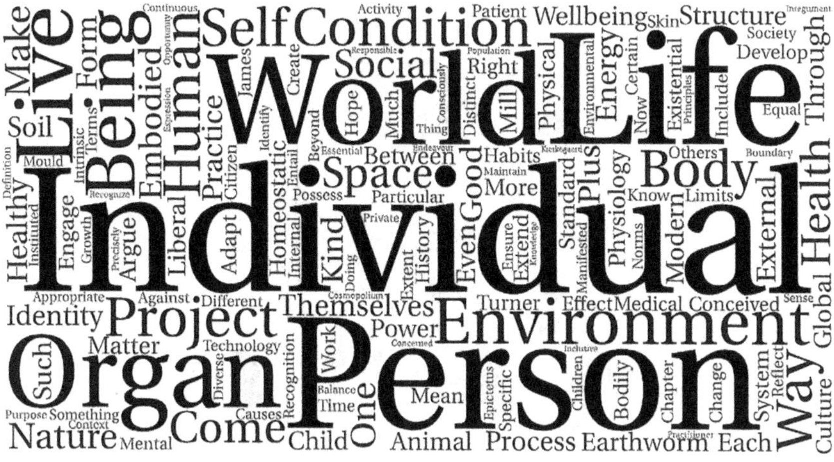

Figure 19.3 Key words relating to Chapter 3.

Source: Author's own work.

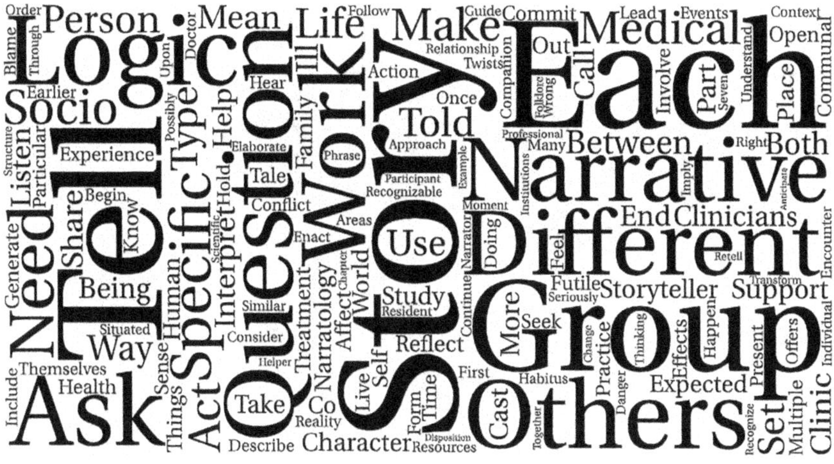

Figure 19.4 Key words relating to Chapter 4.

Source: Author's own work.

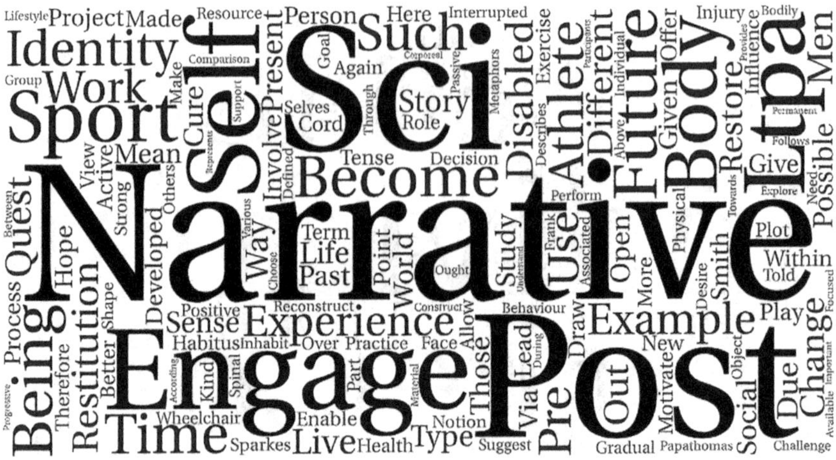

Figure 19.5 Key words relating to Chapter 5.

Source: Author's own work.

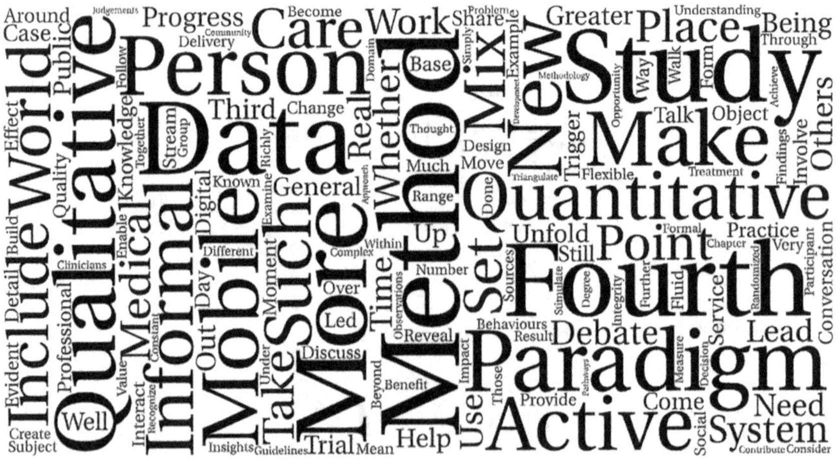

Figure 19.6 Key words relating to Chapter 6.

Source: Authors' own work.

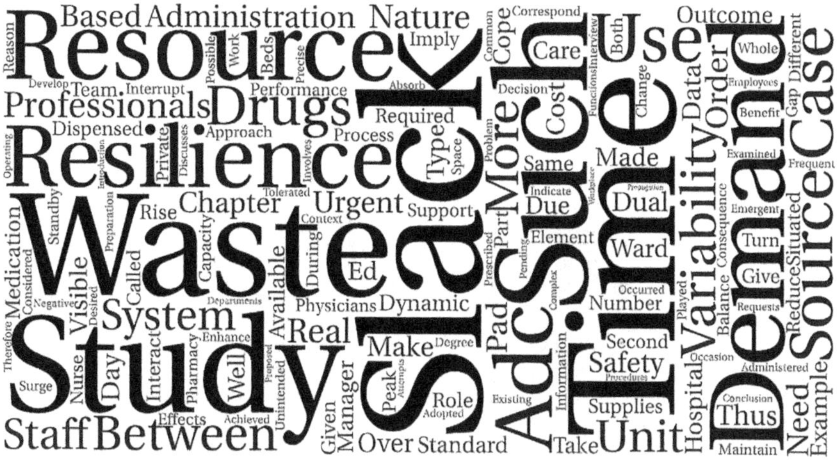

Figure 19.7 Key words relating to Chapter 7.
Source: Authors' own work.

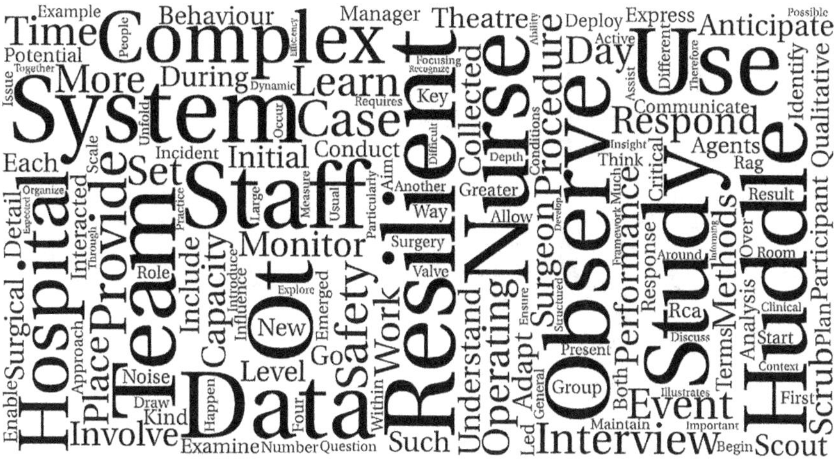

Figure 19.8 Key words relating to Chapter 8.
Source: Authors' own work.

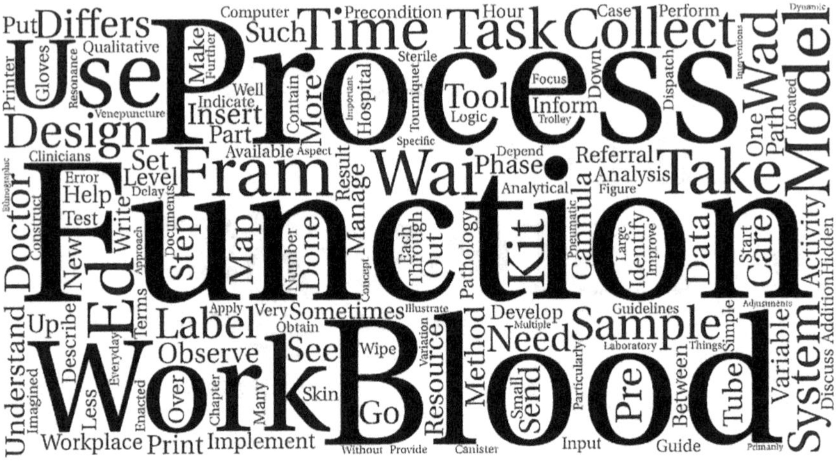

Figure 19.9 Key words relating to Chapter 9.

Source: Authors' own work.

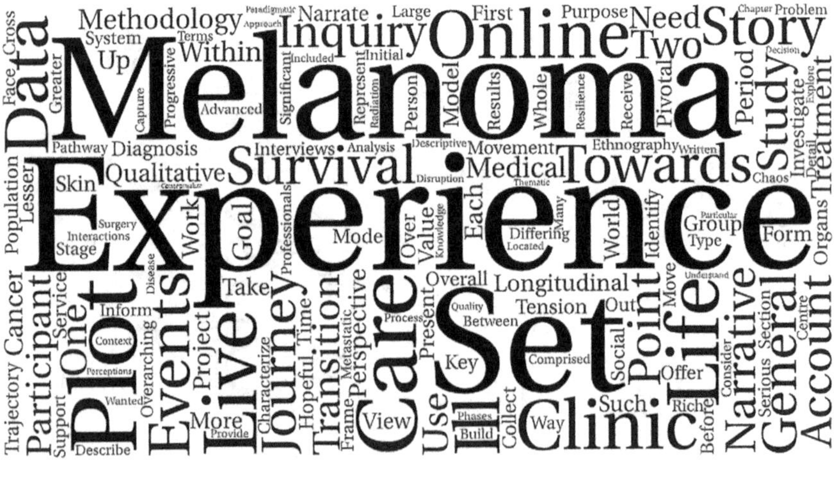

Figure 19.10 Key words relating to Chapter 10.

Source: Authors' own work.

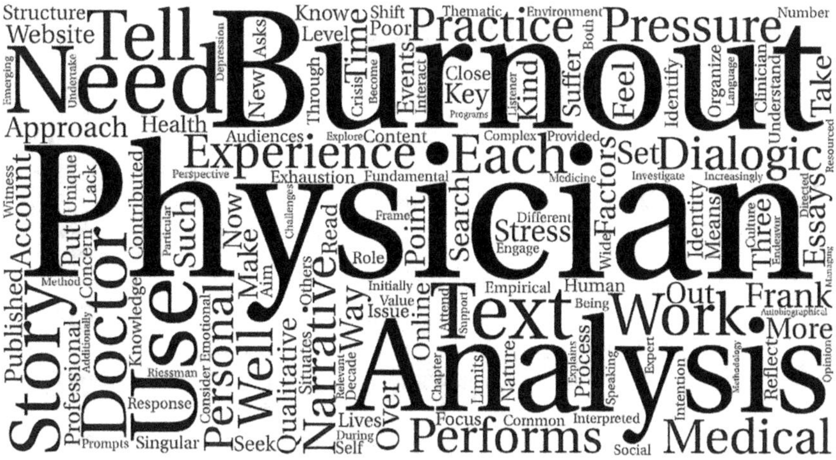

Figure 19.11 Key words relating to Chapter 11.

Source: Authors' own work.

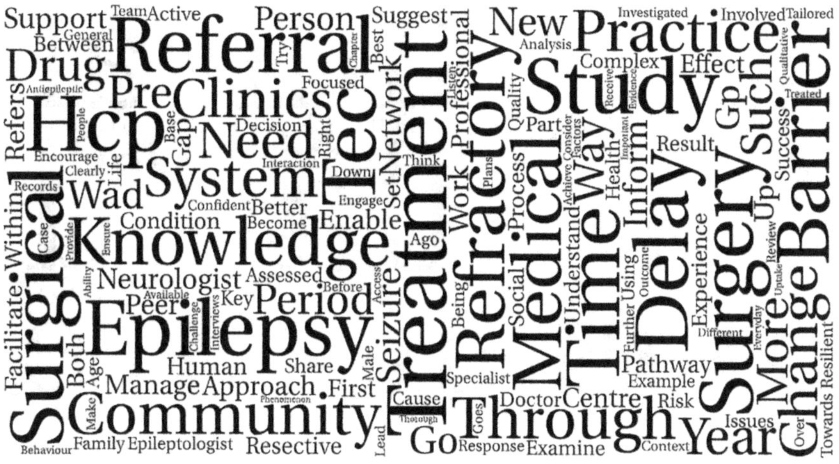

Figure 19.12 Key words relating to Chapter 12.

Source: Authors' own work.

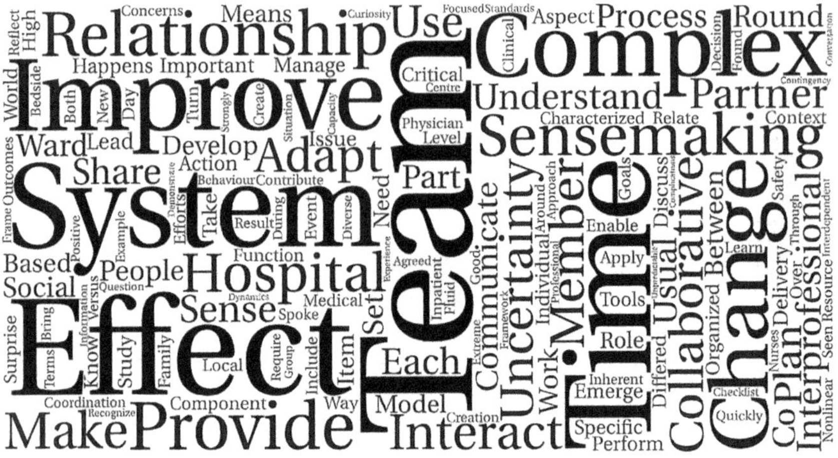

Figure 19.13 Key words relating to Chapter 13.

Source: Authors' own work.

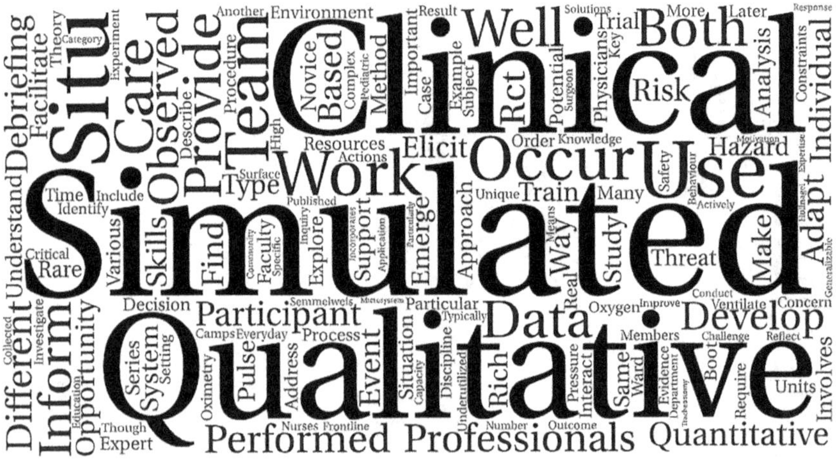

Figure 19.14 Key words relating to Chapter 14.

Source: Authors' own work.

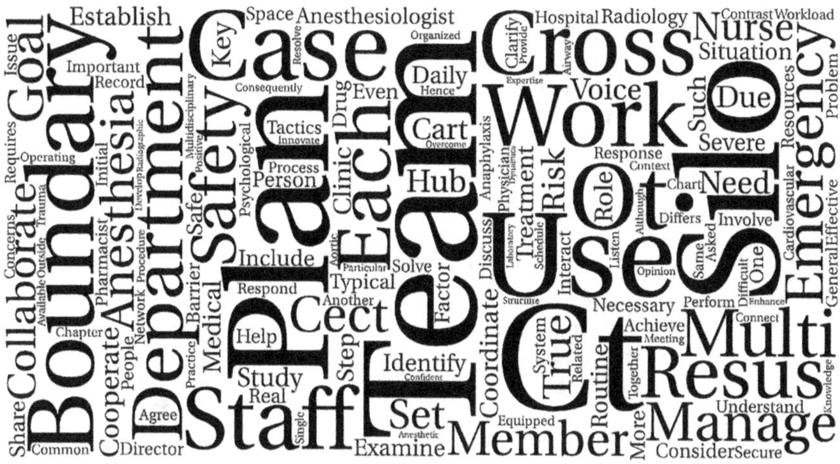

Figure 19.15 Key words relating to Chapter 15.

Source: Authors' own work.

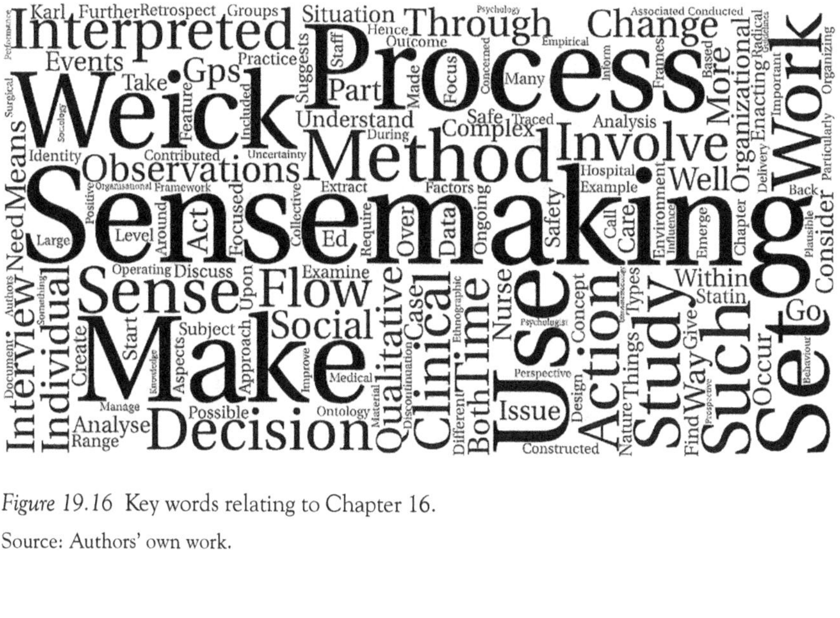

Figure 19.16 Key words relating to Chapter 16.

Source: Authors' own work.

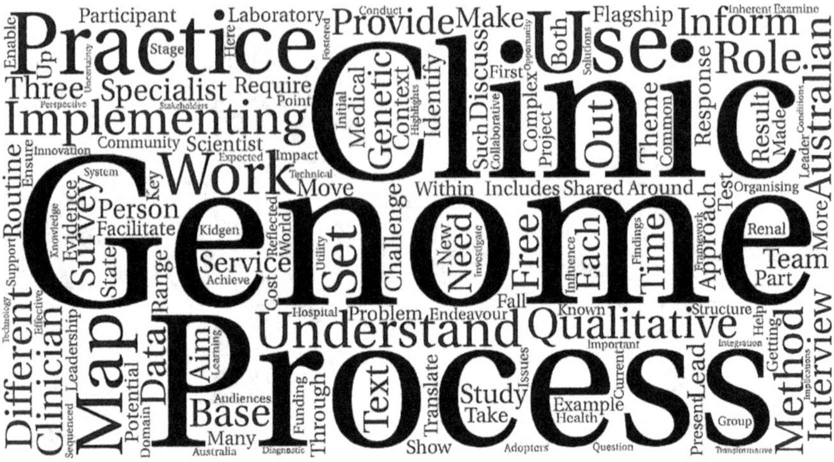

Figure 19.17 Key words relating to Chapter 17.

Source: Authors' own work.

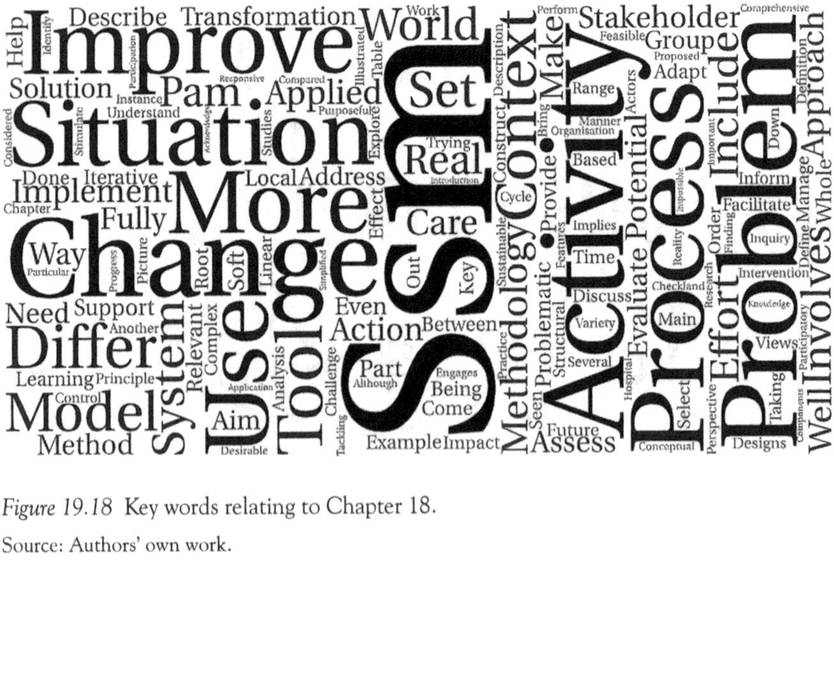

Figure 19.18 Key words relating to Chapter 18.

Source: Authors' own work.

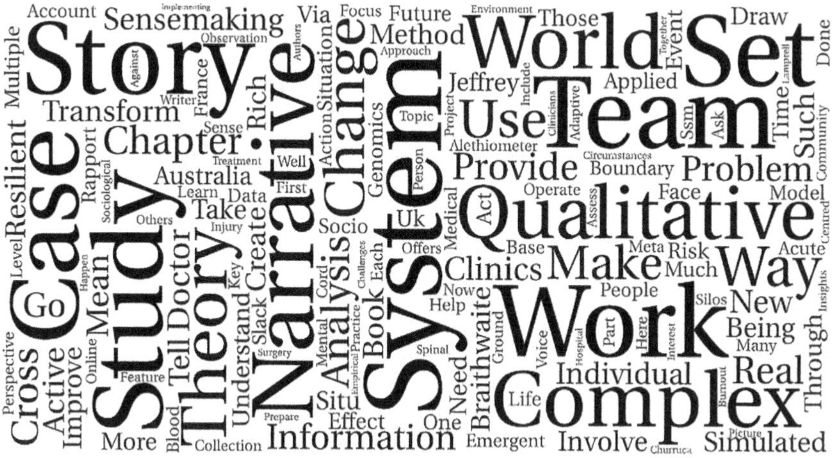

Figure 19.19 Key words relating to Chapter 19.

Source: Authors' own work.

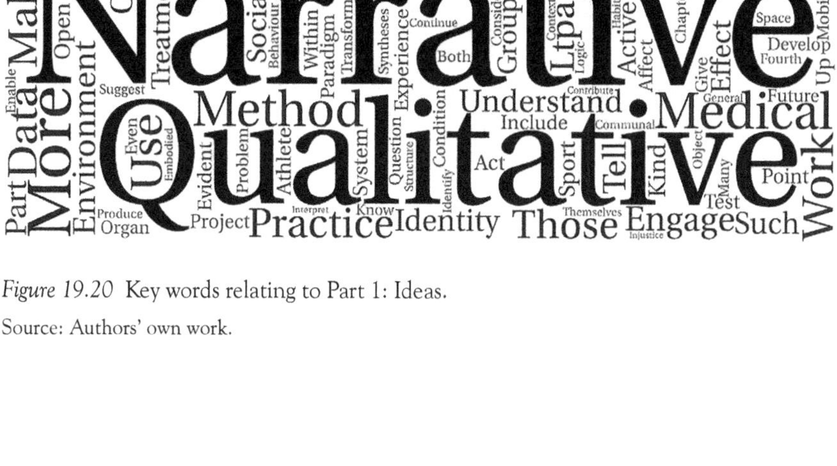

Figure 19.20 Key words relating to Part 1: Ideas.

Source: Authors' own work.

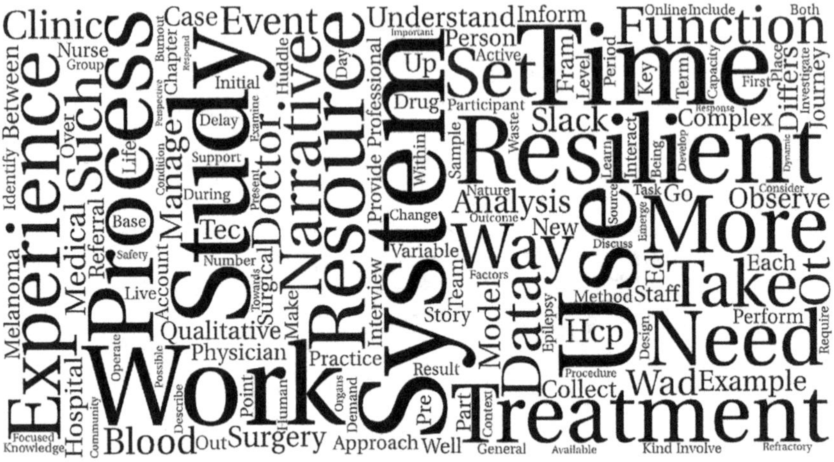

Figure 19.21 Key words relating to Part 2: Systems.

Source: Authors' own work.

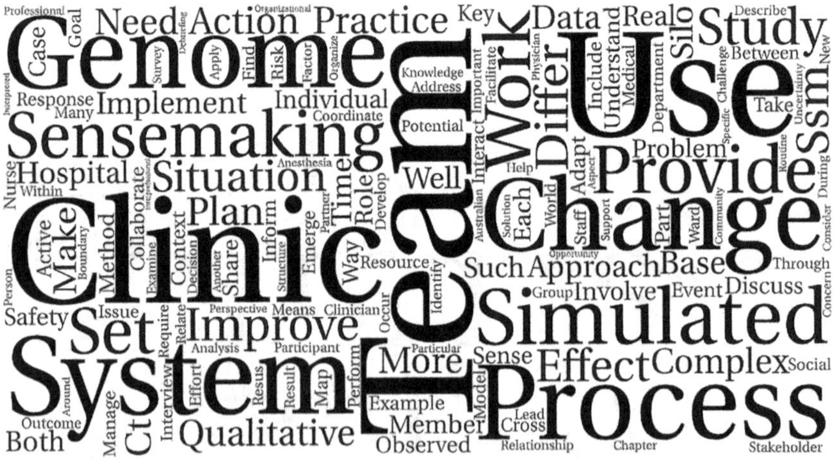

Figure 19.22 Key words relating to Part 3: Solutions.

Source: Authors' own work.

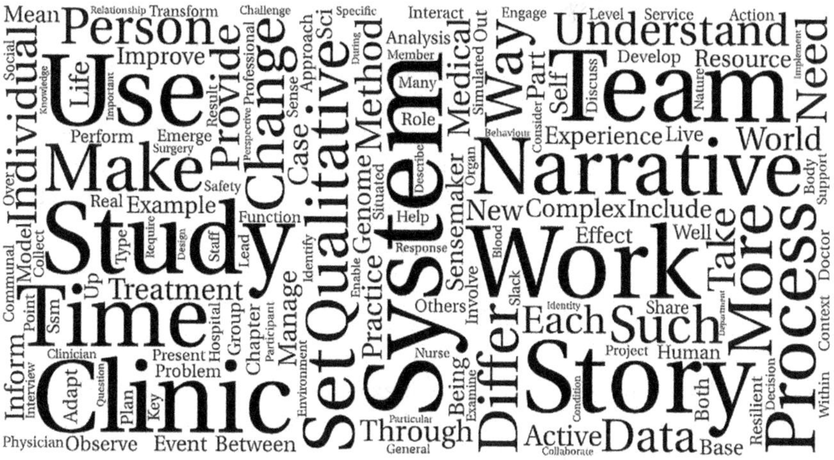

Figure 19.23 Key words relating to Chapters 1–19.

Source: Authors' own work.

them together in scholarly renditions of many aspects of the caring system. We see four key signposts to the future that the book offers.

Signpost 1

Many chapters are a masterclass in explaining *complex ways by which people can, and do, influence, shape or nudge the system in support of transformation.* These range from Britten's qualitative articulation of the voice of the patient; to Mahmoud et al. (this volume) peering into the world of resilience and team huddles in acute settings; to Rapport and Braithwaite applying information developments to understand how research is changing into a fourth paradigm, which can in turn transform care; to Nakamura et al. showing how people can 'meta-team' by crossing boundaries and solving problems in a fluid way; to Lanham et al. illuminating the system via a complexity science frame and an analysis of sensemaking; to Churruca et al. applying Karl Weick's sensemaking idea for guiding change; to Augustsson et al. looking at Soft Systems Methodology (SSM) as a tool for tackling truculent real world problems.

Signpost 2

Others have provided clear *articulations of normally hard-to-unravel theories which can be and are mobilised to explain how the system works or could work better.* The examples we discern here include Saurin et al. using sociotechnical systems theory to understand the power of slack in organisations such that it is seen not as waste but as a buffer for good systems performance, which in turn is needed for system transformation. Lanham et al. and Churruca et al., alongside Mahmoud et al., drawing on complexity theory and anthropologically- and sociologically-grounded theories, each provided a chapter contributing to a better understanding of how care is enacted now. There is a strong use of socio-narrative theories of different hues, too, in the hands of Arthur Frank; Nicky Britten; Andrew C Sparkes; Mary D Patterson and Ellen S Deutsch; and Lamprell and colleagues, which cast a light on the way language and behaviour can be forces for transition, and to act as a catalyst for transformation.

Signpost 3

Yet other chapters have provided us with exemplars or summaries of much that is cutting edge in qualitative empirical findings, and have used their studies to *discuss how healthcare is already transforming, or is on the cusp of transforming*, e.g., Best et al. examining how Australia is preparing for the genomics revolution in the clinic and in practice; Clay-Williams et al. analysing how doctors draw blood, applying the Functional Resonance Analysis Method (FRAM) as a different kind of solution to those normally provided; Shih et al. considering how surgery could be offered in the future to more patients with refractory epilepsy; Patterson and Deutsch, making the case for skills enhancement and team preparation through in situ simulations; and Lamprell et al. in their chapter on the risk of burnout for doctors and the need to care for the carers – and if we do not, then we imperil the very workforce which will provide the transformed care and system we will rely on in the future.

Signpost 4

Another major thrust of the book is to *advocate for patients as transformative agents in healthcare*. That patients can be a catalyst for change also features strongly. The contributions here range from Nigel Rapport, in his chapter articulating individuals and their life-worlds and life-projects; to Arthur Frank, drawing on his work on how storytelling helps patients make sense of the world and how their stories can provide impetus through their socio-narrative perspectives into the health system's consciousness; to Andrew C Sparkes, who continues this longitudinal work of raising narrative to an important level when he analyses spinal cord injury patients; to Lamprell et al., shedding a light on patient narratives of those with melanoma through 214 online patient accounts; and to Nicky Britten, who reminds us that the patient's voice and choices are no less rational than anyone else's and that they should not be seen as less worthy or more subservient. All these writers recognise how crucial it is for patients to have a voice in the care that concerns them.

What this book adds to what we already know

Finally, we want to articulate what the Alethiometer points to for those minded to transform the system or part of it, and what this means to healthcare systems everywhere. Let us use two change models to do this and apply what we have learned about transformation from the book. We can use these models to show how the book's findings can be harnessed in support of that transformation.

First, the Consolidated Framework for Implementation Research (CFIR) is a model that helps guide those who seek to assess implementation by analysing multilevel contexts. It identifies factors that typically influence interventions, implementations and improvement initiatives (Damschroder et al. 2009). A version of this model is in Figure 19.24.

The CFIR draws attention to the factors at work for successful implementation of change – the characteristics of the particular intervention, the inner setting, the outer setting, the individual (or team) characteristics and the processes of change. We can also extend the model as others have done and consider the measures of implementation and the implementation outcomes. We can see the chapters in our book mapping to these CFIR drivers for change. Many show ways to intervene, and detail information about the inner and outer settings.

Intervention	Inner Setting	Outer Setting	Individuals	Process
Adaptability	Structural characteristics	Patient needs and resources	Knowledge and beliefs about intervention	Planning
Trialability	Networks and communication	Cosmopolitan organisation	Self-efficacy	Engaging with opinion leaders, champions etc.
Evidence strength and quality	Culture	Peer pressure	Stage of change	Executing
Intervention source	Implementation climate	External policies and incentives	Identification with the organisation	Reflecting and evaluating
Cost	Readiness for implementation			
Design quality and packaging				

Figure 19.24 Schematic depiction of the Consolidated Framework for Implementation Research (CFIR).

Source: Adapted from Damschroder, LJ, DC Aron, RE Keith, SR Kirsh, JA Alexander, and JC Lowery. 2009. "Fostering implementation of health services research findings into practice: A consolidated framework for advancing implementation science." Implementation Science 4 (50).

More specific examples include Best et al.'s work on the genomic revolution, bringing out the complexities inherent in the processes of adopting genomics throughout Australia. Lamprell et al. discussing medical burnout focus our attention on the individual/team characteristics that can help or hinder intervention success. Clay-Williams et al., in mobilising their FRAM example, focus on measurement of change, but not in the traditional sense of using numbers or statistics. They bring out, via a visual model, a depiction that shows the linked activities ('essential system functions', in FRAM terminology) which go to make up progress, exemplifying how progress can be measured qualitatively over time. And finally Patterson and Deutsch, and Nakamura et al., provide and show qualitative outcomes of different sorts. In Patterson and Deutsch's case this is in the form of simulation-based training and in Nakamura et al.'s chapter it is teaming across boundaries and silos in acute settings. What this all means is that we can map much of the information in the chapters to a change model with strong and widespread application, such as the CFIR.

Second, the key findings of the book, or the models, tools and theories, have to be scaled-up if we are to transform the system or systems. By scaling-up we mean, after demonstrating that change or improvement can be realised in one part of the system, that it is taken elsewhere and enacted in other settings. This is known by similar names although in the hand of experts these often have specific technical meanings – diffusion of innovation, dispersion, dissemination, adoption, take up or spread. Essentially this involves taking a new idea, piece of technology, tool, guideline, method, model of care or piece of evidence and tailoring it each time to the new setting. Figure 19.25 provides a broad outline of a scale-up model (Clay-Williams et al. 2014).

This model envisages that local successful improvements in one context are not necessarily transmitted across healthcare to other contexts unless work is done to enable that transmission. In scaling-up, the change to be shared across a system must have some active ingredients to enable the successful spread.

Typically, this is some level of agency which enables the change or evidence to be received, embraced or facilitated in other settings. For instance, Augustsson et al.'s SSM tool would need to become more widely known, and its benefits demonstrated to a broader range of people, for it to be more accepted across healthcare. Similarly, Nicky Britten made the case that a deeper understanding by health professionals of the real world experiences of patients could lead to productive improvement in services to those patients. Yet this would require more widespread acceptance by health professionals treating them, and greater levels of health literacy and advocacy amongst patient populations.

Furthermore, according to the work of Nigel Rapport, Arthur Frank and Andrew C Sparkes, the level of agency and respect for individual autonomy and decision-making would need to change, with greater dialogue between patients, healthcare professionals, system designers, managers and health policy implementers if we are to ensure agency is more firmly placed in the hands of those receiving care. Most importantly, in this respect, agency would need to be more fully recognised as an individualistic concept, a person-centred 'project'. Transmitting improvement

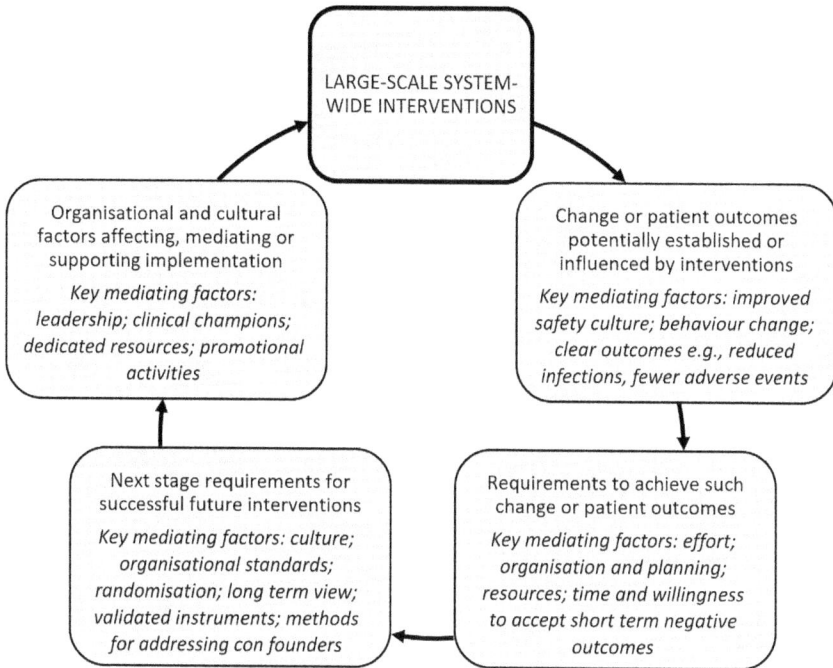

Figure 19.25 Factors affecting, and affected by, large scale system-wide interventions for implementation success and system transformation.

Source: ® Reprinted with permission from Springer Nature: BioMed Central Ltd. BMC Health Services Research. Clay-Williams, R, H Nosrati, FC Cunningham, K Hillman, and J Braithwaite. "Do large-scale hospital-and system-wide interventions improve patient outcomes: A systematic review." *BMC Health Services Research* 14 (369), CC BY 2.0 (2014).

across healthcare to other contexts through scaling-up could, therefore, ensure an active ingredient of reflection is placed on personal narratives and the role of narrative storytelling in uncovering personhood, to drive patient advocacy forward. As with professional autonomy, patient narratives are invaluable for understanding patient need and experience, while together with professional autonomy, they offer the potential for new symbiotic relationships that drive professional decision-making forward during care processes and inform patient care journeys.

Conclusion

Four signposts – Alethiometer-inspired navigation aids – point the way to the transformed healthcare system and are represented by methods to influence, shape or nudge the system; theories to explain how the system works or can work better; aspects of the system already transforming or about to do so; and the activation of patients as transformative agents; completes our work in this book. Implementation success and scaleup of that success are two important pre-conditions that we have added. These are mechanisms for taking the ideas, tools, theories and evidence from the book's chapters to support transformational activities.

In the end, we believe there is something in the book for everyone interested in better care for more people. Whether we want to transform healthcare by leveraging patient power in the mould of Andrew C Sparkes, Arthur Frank, Nigel Rapport or Nicky Britten, or exploit ideas such as resilient healthcare (Mahmoud et al. this volume; Patterson and Deutsch this volume), understand systems' properties such as slack (Saurin and Ferreira this volume) and complexity (Augustsson et al. this volume), map patient trajectories (Lamprell et al. this volume; Shih et al. this volume) and word-as-done (Clay-Williams et al. this volume), care for carers (Lamprell et al. this volume), enable effective teamwork (Nakamura et al. this volume), facilitate peoples' sensemaking (Lanham et al. this volume; Churruca et al. this volume) or revolutionize the way care is delivered (Best et al. this volume), we have documented here a plethora of gateways to an improved, reformed or transformed system.

As both contributors and editors, we think there is much to celebrate, learn and inspire in these pages. We hope you do too.

References

Augustsson, H, K Churruca, and J Braithwaite. This volume. "Much more than old wine in new bottles: Soft systems methodology (SSM) for healthcare improvement." In *Transforming Healthcare with Qualitative Research*, edited by F Rapport and J Braithwaite. Oxford: Routledge.

Best, S, JC Long, E McPherson, N Taylor, and J Braithwaite. This volume. "Deep inside the genomics revolution: On the frontlines of care." In *Transforming Healthcare with Qualitative Research*, edited by F Rapport and J Braithwaite. Oxford: Routledge.

Britten, N. This volume "Qualitative evidence synthesis and conceptual development." In *Transforming Healthcare with Qualitative Research*, edited by F Rapport and J Braithwaite. Oxford: Routledge.

Churruca, K, LA Ellis, JC Long, and J Braithwaite. This volume. "'What on earth is going on and what should I do now?' Sensemaking as a qualitative process." In *Transforming Healthcare with Qualitative Research*, edited by F Rapport and J Braithwaite. Oxford: Routledge.

Clay-Williams, R, E Austin, J Braithwaite, and E Hollnagel. This volume. "Qualitative assessment to improve everyday activities: Work-as-imagined and work-as-done." In *Transforming Healthcare with Qualitative Research*, edited by F Rapport and J Braithwaite. Oxford: Routledge.

Clay-Williams, R, H Nosrati, FC Cunningham, K Hillman, and J Braithwaite. 2014. "Do large-scale hospital-and system-wide interventions improve patient outcomes: A systematic review." *BMC Health Services Research* 14 (369).

Damschroder, LJ, DC Aron, RE Keith, SR Kirsh, JA Alexander, and JC Lowery. 2009. "Fostering implementation of health services research findings into practice: A consolidated framework for advancing implementation science." *Implementation Science* 4 (50).

Frank, AW. This volume. "Socio-narratology and the clinical encounter between human beings." In *Transforming Healthcare with Qualitative Research*, edited by F Rapport and J Braithwaite. Oxford: Routledge.

Frank, AW. 2012. "Practicing dialogical narrative analysis." In *Varieties of Narrative Analysis*, edited by JA Holstein and JF Gubrium. Thousand Oaks: Sage.

Lamprell, K, F Rapport, and J Braithwaite. This volume. "Look the other way: Patient-centred care begins with care for our physicians. A dialogic narrative analysis of three personal essays." In *Transforming Healthcare with Qualitative Research*, edited by F Rapport and J Braithwaite. Oxford: Routledge.

Lamprell, K, F Rapport, and J Braithwaite. This volume. "Narrativising cancer patients' longitudinal experiences of care: Qualitative inquiry into lived and online melanoma stories." In *Transforming Healthcare with Qualitative Research*, edited by F Rapport and J Braithwaite. Oxford: Routledge.

Lanham, HJ, JA Pugh, DC Aron, and LK Leykum. This volume. "Sensemaking as a strategy for managing uncertainty: Change and surprise in hospital settings." In *Transforming Healthcare with Qualitative Research*, edited by F Rapport and J Braithwaite. Oxford: Routledge.

Mahmoud, Z, K Churruca, LA Ellis, R Clay-Williams, and J Braithwaite. This volume. "Using qualitative methods to understand resilience in complex systems." In *Transforming Healthcare with Qualitative Research*, edited by F Rapport and J Braithwaite. Oxford: Routledge.

Nakamura, K, S Nakajima, T Abe, and K Nakajima. This volume. "Cross-boundary teaming to establish resilience among isolated 'Silos'." In *Transforming Healthcare with Qualitative Research*, edited by F Rapport and J Braithwaite. Oxford: Routledge.

Patterson, MD, and ES Deutsch. This volume. "Simulation to solve health system problems." In *Transforming Healthcare with Qualitative Research*, edited by F Rapport and J Braithwaite. Oxford: Routledge.

Pullman, P. 2011. *His Dark Materials*. 3rd ed. London: Scholastic. Original edition, Northern lights, 1995, The subtle knife, 1997, The amber spyglass, 2000.

Rapport, F, and J Braithwaite. This volume. "The fourth research paradigm: Activating researchers for real world need." In *Transforming Healthcare with Qualitative Research*, edited by F Rapport and J Braithwaite. Oxford: Routledge.

Rapport, N. This volume "The life-project of personal wellbeing: Modern healthcare and the individuality of health." In *Transforming Healthcare with Qualitative Research*, edited by F Rapport and J Braithwaite. Oxford: Routledge.

Saurin, TA, and DMC Ferreira. This volume. "Slack resources in healthcare systems: Waste or resilience?" In *Transforming Healthcare with Qualitative Research*, edited by F Rapport and J Braithwaite. Oxford: Routledge.

Shih, P, F Rapport, JC Long, E Francis-Auton, M Bierbaum, M Faris, and R Clay-Williams. This volume. "Resilient healthcare in refractory epilepsy treatment: Illuminating successful people-centred patient care." In *Transforming Healthcare with Qualitative Research*, edited by F Rapport and J Braithwaite. Oxford: Routledge.

Sparkes, AC. "Interrupted body projects and the narrative reconstruction of self." In *Transforming Healthcare with Qualitative Research*, edited by F Rapport and J Braithwaite. Oxford: Routledge.

Weick, KE. 1995. *Sensemaking in Organizations*. Vol. 3. Thousand Oaks: Sage.

Word Art. 2019. https://wordart.com/create.

Index

For Product Safety Concerns and Information please contact our EU
representative GPSR@taylorandfrancis.com
Taylor & Francis Verlag GmbH, Kaufingerstraße 24, 80331 München, Germany